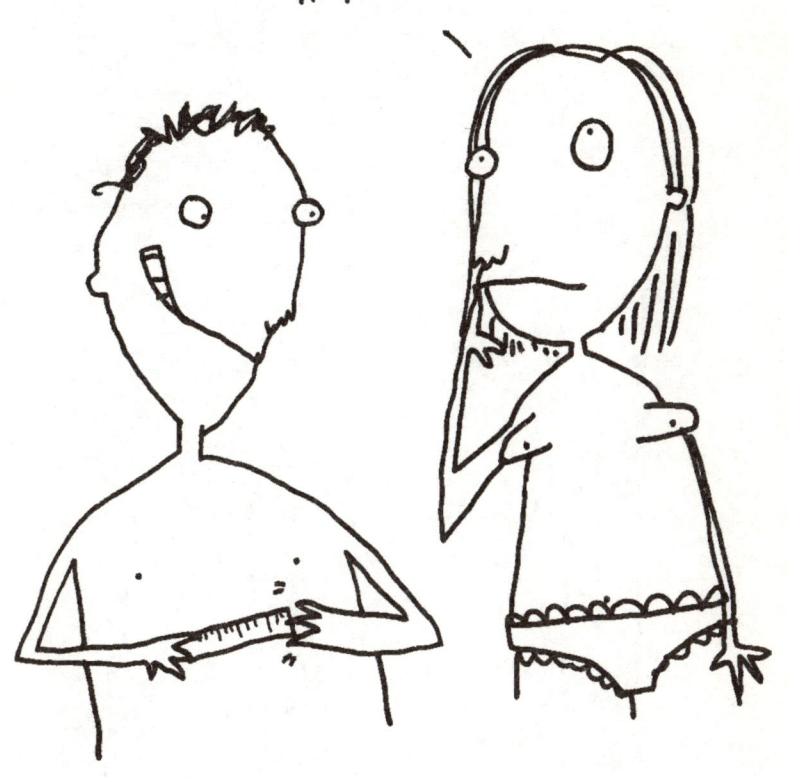

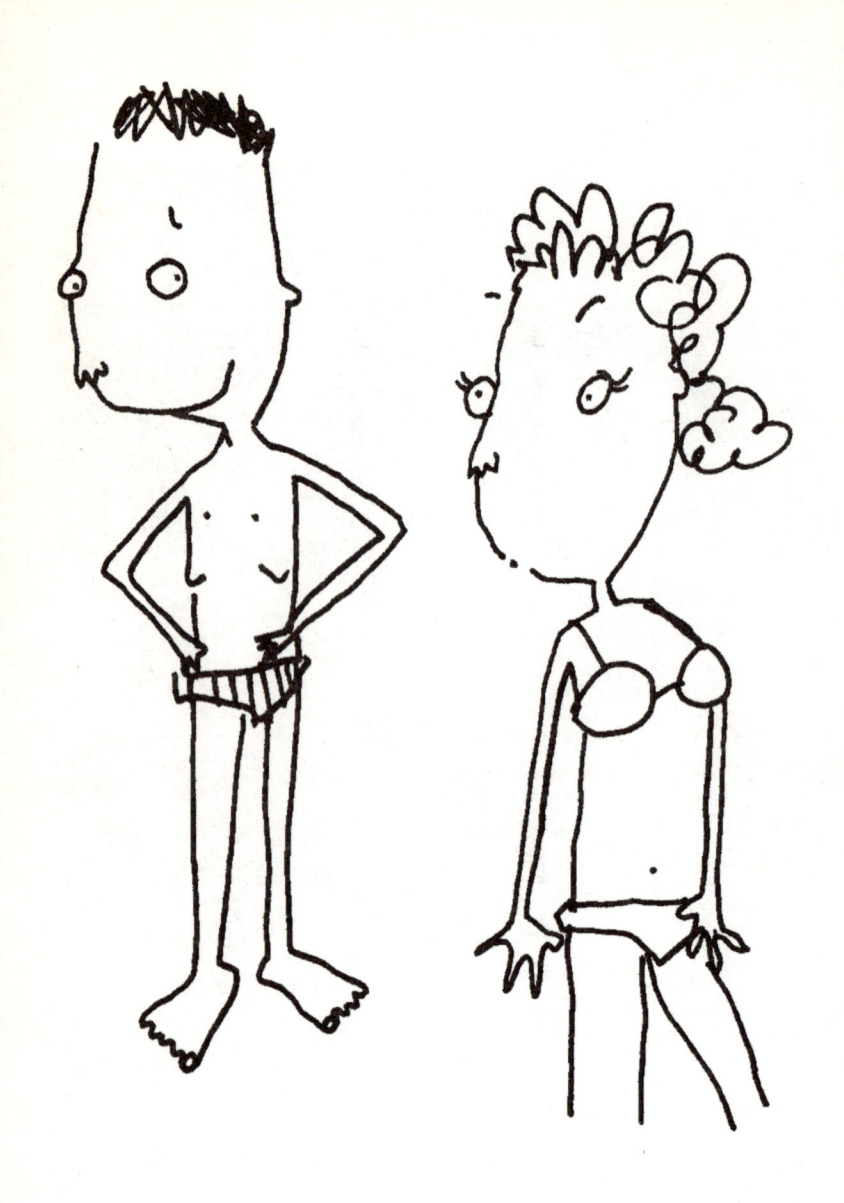

ADAM vs. Eve

THIS IS A CARLTON BOOK

Text, illustrations and design copyright © 2004
Carlton Books Limited

This edition published by
Carlton Books Limited 2004
20 Mortimer Street
London W1T 3JW

This book is sold subject to the condition that it shall not, by way of trade or otherwise, be lent, resold, hired out or otherwise circulated without the publisher's prior written consent in any form of cover or binding other than that in which it is published and without a similar condition including this condition being imposed upon the subsequent purchaser.

All rights reserved
A CIP catalogue record for this book is
available from the British Library

ISBN 1 84442 647 5

executive editor: Lisa Dyer
senior art editor: Zoë Dissell
designer: Diane Spender
copy editors: Lol Henderson and Lara Maiklem
production controller: Caroline Alberti
illustrators: Sarah Nayler and Adam Wright

Printed and bound in Great Britain

CARLTON BOOKS

ADAM vs. Eve

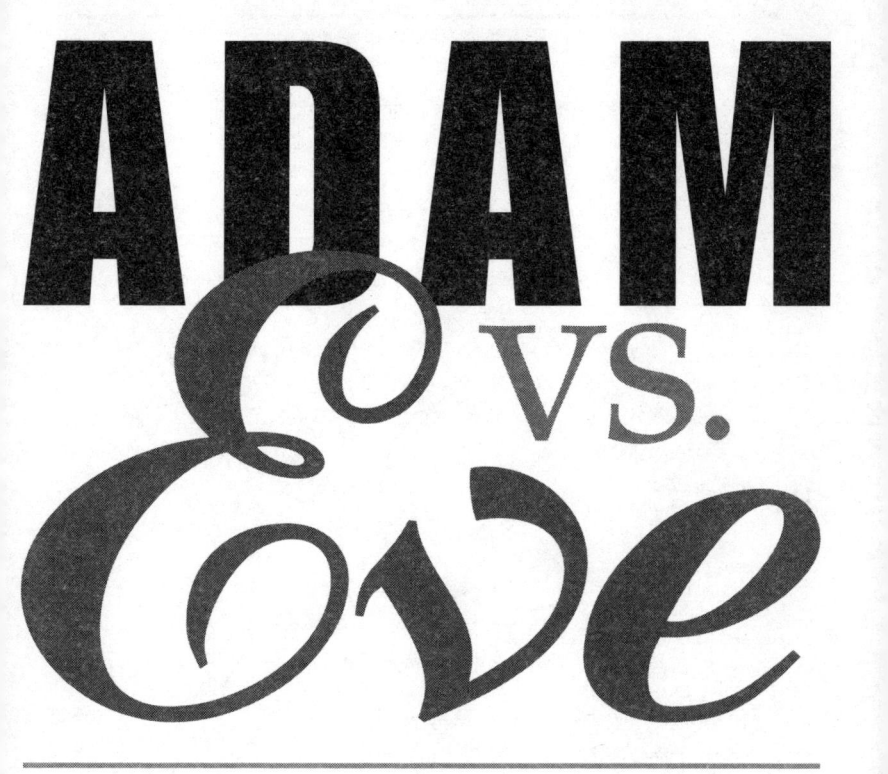

jokes from the frontline in the battle of the sexes

paul rogan and **justin rosenholtz**

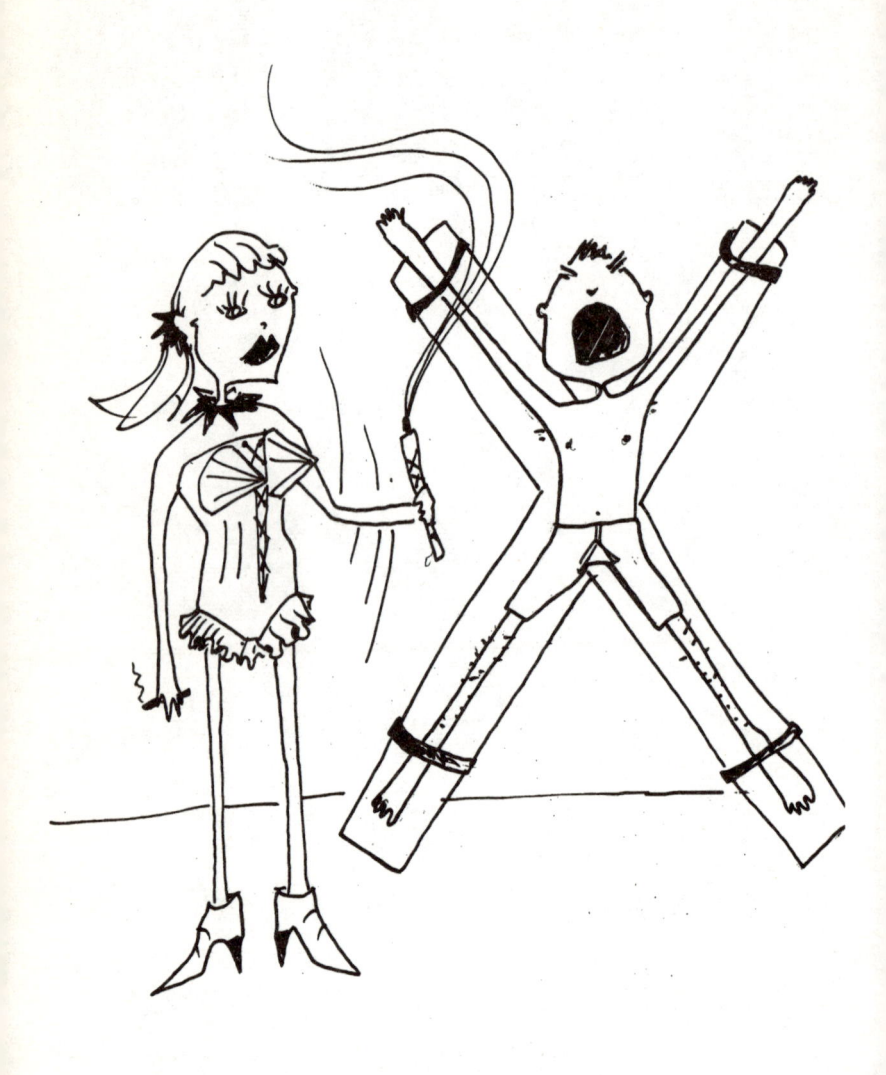

Contents

1 The Dating Game **9**

2 In the Bedroom **31**

3 Going Places Together **47**

4 Tying the Knot **63**

5 Domestic Bliss **79**

6 Advice for the Sexes **95**

7 Diary of a Relationship **113**

8 Breaking up is Hard to Do **121**

9 Growing Old Disgracefully **129**

10 And Finally ...
Some Jokes to Share **139**

CHAPTER ONE

The Dating Game

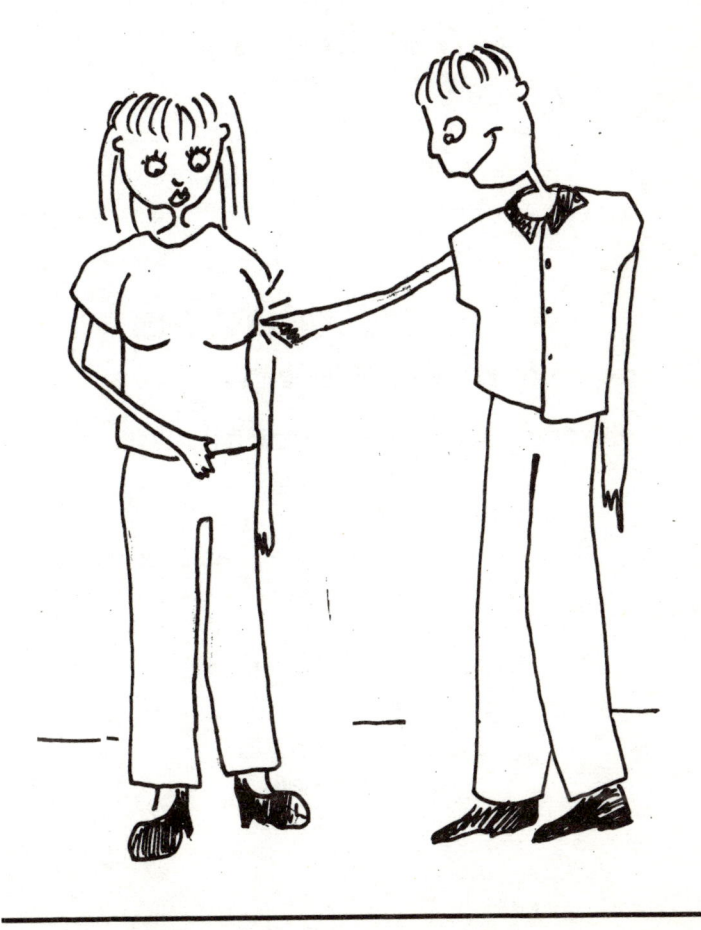

Good places to meet **men**:

Will readings.
Charity fundraisers.
Fires.
Fire stations.
Bars where **firemen** go.
Polo matches.
Tiffany's.
The Oscars.
Monte Carlo.

Bad places to meet **men**:

On the floor of the **men's room** in a gay bar.
Parole hearings.
Anger management classes.
Sex addiction counseling sessions.
Pawnbrokers.
A carjacking.
Star Trek conventions.
A holding center at Guantanamo Bay.
Bankruptcy courts.
Sperm banks.
Key West.

Good places
to meet women:

Nurses' residences.
Low self-esteem workshops.
Sex addiction clinics.
The funeral of their wealthy husband.
Cheerleading tryouts.
Chick flicks.
Porn film awards.
Justin Timberlake concerts.
Breast implant centers.
Sweden.

Bad places to meet women:

VD clinics.
Shopaholics anonymous meetings.
Needle exchange programs.
k.d. lang gigs.
Andrea Dworkin seminars.
Open day at a convent.
Take Back the Night marches.
A therapist's waiting room.
Chicken Ranch **Brothel**, Nevada.
Crack houses.
Bangkok.

Great six-pack

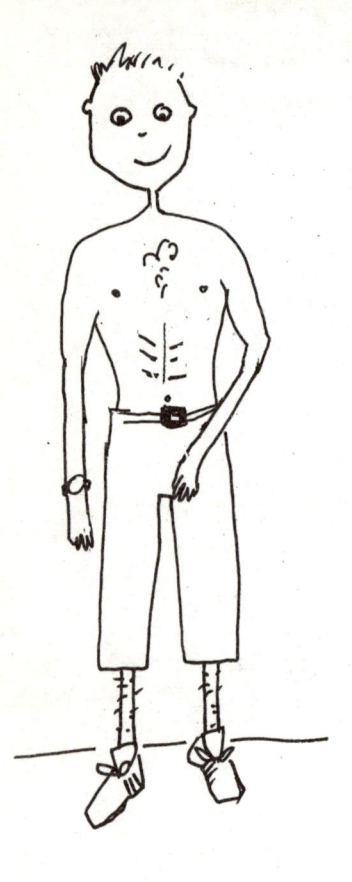

Bad six-pack

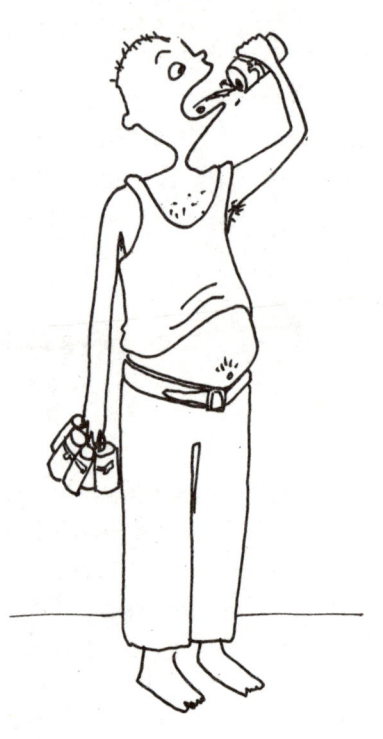

13 • THE DATING GAME

Great rack

Bad rack

A man is about to go on a **blind date**. He's having cold feet and phones his best friend. "What the hell am I supposed to do if it turns out that **she's ugly**?" he asks. "I'll have to spend the whole evening with her!"

His friend tries to calm him down: "Look, why don't you just go and pick her up, and see what she looks like before you decide anything. **Maybe she'll be really good-looking, and you'll be fine.** But if you don't like what you're seeing, all you have to do is shout 'Aaaaauuurghhhh!' and pretend to have an asthma attack."

"That's a great plan," says the guy, and sets off for the date. He knocks on the girl's door and when she opens it, he is relieved and delighted to see that she is **stunningly beautiful and sexy**.

He is just about to say hello when she suddenly shouts: **"Aaaaauuurghhhh!"**

How a **woman** gets ready for a date:

Select, dress, review, undress, **redress**, consult, discuss, shop, redress, freak-out, return, reselect, redress, **panic**, accessorize, preen, depart. Return, change shoes, depart.

How a **man** gets ready for a date:

Sniff underarms, depart.

Perfect opening lines a **woman** wants to hear:

- Hi, I'm George Clooney.
- Hello, I need a beautiful woman to make my yacht look perfect.
- I'm a lawyer, and I earn **six figures a year.**
- I'm ready for a committed relationship.
- You combine chic fashion sense with a gift for accessorizing.
- I find cellulite sexy.
- They need me at the Fire Station, but can I have your number?
- I've got a **discount at Gucci**.
- I have all the qualities women admire in gay men—but I'm straight.
- I can give you head until you beg for mercy.

Perfect opening lines a **man** wants to hear:

- I'm drunk.
- **I'm not wearing underwear.**
- I have very low expectations.
- I find beer guts sexy.
- I'm easy and I don't expect you to call me the next day.
- I admire men who can come in less than two minutes.
- Can we watch the football after?
- Will you help me **soap my breasts?**
- I like the taste of an unwashed penis.
- My twin sister fancies you too—and we're both from Sweden.

How to tell if the date's going well **for him:**

1. Mid-date she changes into lingerie.

2. She hasn't rolled her eyes during your interesting discourse on digital recording formats.

3. She didn't seem suspicious when you lied about your salary.

4. Her life story didn't make you feel nauseous.

5. When she had **spinach in her teeth** you thought it was cute.

6. She doesn't remind you of your mother.

7. She's smiling, but without the telltale glazed look of Prozac.

8. She orders steak and fries and clears her plate.

9. She's BLOWING you under the table.

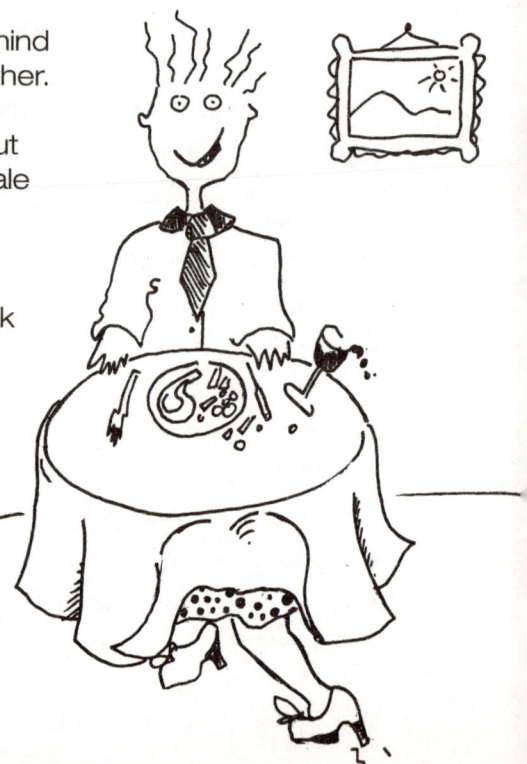

How to tell if the date's going well **for her:**

1. He admires your shoes.

2. He nodded, smiled, and listened during your tale of That Bitch At Work.

3. He says the gorgeous waitress is **"too skinny."**

4. He tells you about the new book he's written: *Cunnilingus, the Expert's Guide*.

5. When you admire his Rolex, he gives it to you.

6. He brings glowing letters of recommendation from his previous girlfriends.

7. Women in the restaurant keep asking if he's George Clooney.

8. He tells you your cold sore "adds character."

9. He says he thinks spring weddings are romantic.

The advice column

DEAR ADVICE COLUMN,

I AM, IF I DO SAY SO MYSELF, A VERY GOOD-LOOKING MAN. NOT TO BRAG, BUT I'M A BABE MAGNET. MY PROBLEM IS MY GIRLFRIEND. SHE IS SMART AND FUNNY AND REALLY COOL, BUT TO BE FRANK, SHE IS NOT THAT ATTRACTIVE. I LOVE HER AND HAVE NEVER MET SOMEONE I'D RATHER BE WITH MORE, BUT SOMETIMES HER LOOKS BOTHER ME.

SIGNED HANDSOME AND KNOWS IT

Dear Handsome and Knows It,

There has never been, in the history of the world, a couple where the man is better-looking than the woman. We're sorry, but you must dump her for someone prettier. She'll understand.

Dear Advice Column,

I am a beautiful woman and I can get any man I want. I love my boyfriend: he's kind and he treats me better than any man I've ever met. The thing is, he's not that attractive; in fact he's quite unattractive. It shouldn't matter, but I can't help it.

Signed Perfect-looking

Dear Perfect-looking,

What is the problem here? You have a wonderful man who treats you well. It is what's inside that counts. You should be ashamed of yourself for being so superficial.

Dicktionary

He says	He means
I'll call you.	I won't call you.
I'll definitely call you.	Maybe I will, maybe I won't.
I'll call you Tuesday at seven.	I have a date with a hot blonde on Monday and I'll see how that goes.

Dic**she**nary

She says	She means
Call me.	I haven't had a date since 1998.
Definitely call me.	I'm desperate and I have no self-esteem.
Call me Tuesday at seven.	How did the date with the blonde go?

How to tell if the date's going badly **for him**:

1. She keeps thanking Jesus for sending her a man.

2. She says she doesn't like the restaurant as it isn't macrobiotic.

3. She's **brought her lawyer "to observe."**

4. She's flirting with the waiter within five minutes.

5. She asks you to sign a Pre-Prandial Agreement.

6. A timer keeps going off to remind her to take her medication.

7. She keeps taking phone calls from a "Doug."

8. When asked about her previous boyfriends, she talks evasively about how unfair restraining orders are.

9. She keeps calling her AA sponsor to discuss how the date is going.

10. She asks whether you have any photos or mementos so she can build a shrine.

How to tell if the date's going badly **for her**:

1. He said he was going to the bathroom but he's been gone for 20 minutes and he took his coat.

2. He's aggressively asking the guy at the next table, "Are you looking at my woman?"

3. The date is at McDonalds and he wants you to pay half the bill.

4. The waitress has slipped him her number, and so has the woman at the next table.

5. All night long, women come over to your table and slap him.

6. He's spent all evening **prodding your breasts and asking, "Are those real?"**

7. He says no woman will ever compare to his school French teacher.

8. He orders you a Vodka and Rohypnol.

9. He suggests a threesome with you and the waitress.

10. After dinner he says, "On my signal, and when the waiter's not looking, RUN!"

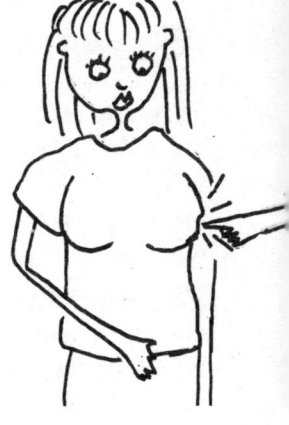

The "How many people have you slept with before me?" ready reckoner:

To find out the true number of women he has slept with, take the number he tells you and divide by three.

To find out the **true number** of men **she** has slept with, **multiply by three.**

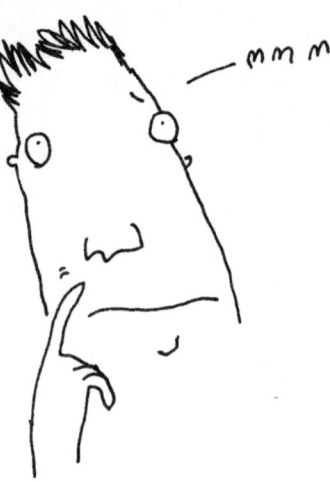

A man goes to a bar and sees a very attractive woman sitting by herself. Being a shy type, he has to pluck up courage to approach her, so after a couple of drinks he goes up to her, and says, quietly and politely: "Excuse me, I noticed you were here by yourself. I wonder if you would mind if I joined you."

She turns to look at him and shouts, **"NO, there's no way I'll have sex with YOU!"**

Everybody in the bar turns to look at them. The man walks back to his table, completely embarrassed and crushed. Shortly afterwards, the man is putting on his coat to leave when he notices the woman approaching him. She sits down, smiles a wry smile and says, "Look, I'm really sorry if I embarrassed you just now. I'm doing a Ph.D. in Psychology and testing peoples' reactions to embarrassing situations."

He smiles back at her, stands up and shouts, **"What do you mean, $300 for the night?"**

Dicktionary

He says	**He means**
You look nice.	I can see your nipples.
I like your house.	When can I move in and not pay rent?
I like your roommate.	Why didn't I meet her first?

Dic**she**nary

She says	**She means**
I like your tie.	Once we're a couple that's the first thing that goes.
We should go now, I have an early start.	Date's over pal.
I've been looking forward to this.	I've been obsessing about what our children will look like.

Her pick-up line comebacks:

Can I buy you a drink?
I'd rather have the cash.

Hey babe, how do you like your eggs in the morning?
Unfertilized by you, pal.

Do you have any Irish in you? Would you like some?
Why? Do you know Pierce Brosnan?

Your place or mine?
His.

You've got great breasts
So have you (unfortunately, they're not as big as yours).

Cheer up darling, it may never happen.
It just has.

May I have the pleasure of this dance?
No, I'd like some pleasure, too.

When should I phone you?
Well, I'm not in tomorrow so call me then.

Would you like a drink?
Do you really think our relationship will last that long?

Have you ever done it with a real man?
No, why have you?

If Brad Pitt doesn't turn up, I'll be waiting over there.
If Brad Pitt does turn up, I'll send him over.

Nice pair of legs, when do they open?
Way after your bedtime.

Get your coat—you've scored.
You're right, I'm leaving with him.

Come and sit on my lap and we'll talk about the first thing that pops up.
No thanks, I don't like small talk.

Hey babe, want to get lucky?
Judging from your face, it doesn't look like you were.

If I said you had a beautiful body, would you hold it against me?
If I told you I had a gun, would you hold it against your head and pull the trigger?

Do you believe in one-night stands?
Normally yes, but for you I'll make an exception.

His pick-up line
comebacks:

May I introduce myself?
Sure—try those people over there.

Is it hot in here or is it just you?
It's hot.

Kiss me.
You'll have to drug me first.

Please talk to me so that creep over there will leave me alone.
I just said that to someone about you.

Where have you been all my life?
What do you mean? I wasn't even born for the first half of it.

I'm sure I've noticed you before.
I'm not sure I've even noticed you yet.

How old are you?
25. Add that to your IQ and you might reach three figures.

I can fulfill your sexual fantasy.
Cool! Is Pamela Anderson here?

My ideal man has a great sense of humor.
Well, he'd need one.

You must be tired 'cause you've been running through my mind all night.
Yes, but unfortunately I couldn't escape.

Do you believe in love at first sight?
No, but after seeing you I believe in the Loch Ness Monster.

I think **you're** the cutest guy here tonight.
That's why I think I can do better than you.

Blind Date Conversations

For him:

Do say: Hi, I'm Ted.
Don't say: No, I've never heard of Ted, me no speaky English.

Do say: Your friend says you have a big personality.
Don't say: Although your friend didn't mention the big wart on the side of your nose.

Do say: I'm just going to find a table for us.
Don't say: I'm just … going.

Do say: Would you like a drink?
Don't say: Maybe you'll be more attractive when I'm smashed out of my head.

Do say: I'm pleased to meet you.
Don't say: I don't care what you look like, I haven't had sex for two years.

Do say: I'm very pleased to meet you.
Don't say: Damn! You're much better-looking than me. Guess you'll be making your excuses soon.

Do say: Mary! What a surprise!
Don't say: Some idiot has set me up with my ex-girlfriend from Hell.

For her:

Do say: I didn't recognize you from your description.
Don't say: Because the description didn't say "squat and ugly."

Do say: I hear you have quite a sense of humor.
Don't say: Your description of yourself is the biggest joke **EVER**.

Do say: I'm told you have many attractive qualities.
Don't say: Although attractiveness isn't one of them.

Do say: I didn't know you had dark hair.
Don't say: ... growing out of your nose and ears.

Do say: Everyone says we'll have so much in common.
Don't say: What the hell must everyone think of me?

Do say: I'm pleased to meet you.
Don't say: I'm desperate for a date for my younger sister's wedding.

Do say: Oh, I see you've arrived straight from work in your uniform.
Don't say: No one told me you were a fucking janitor!

CHAPTER TWO

2

In the Bedroom

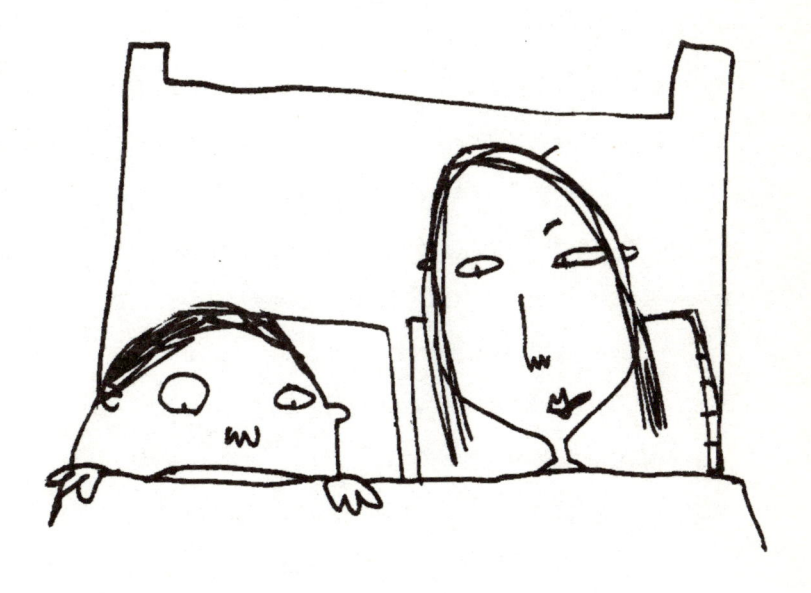

Her idea of a sexual fantasy...

I'm alone in my hotel room in Hawaii, naked on the huge, Egyptian cotton-covered bed. The heat is powerful. There's a knock on the door. "Room service," calls the deep, manly voice from outside. I pull on a La Perla slip and call him in. It's **George Clooney**, carrying a tray of champagne. I say, "Aren't you George Clooney?" He says, "Yeah, I'm researching the part of a waiter for a movie." He pours the champagne. "Have one for yourself," I say. He says, "A toast to you, the most beautiful woman in Hawaii." I say, "You're pretty damn beautiful yourself." He leans over and kisses me. I taste the champagne on his mouth. He kisses my neck and strokes my hair, and works his way down my body, with gentle, caressing kisses. I feel his hardness against me.

I reach for the zipper...

His idea of a sexual fantasy...

Some babe with big tits bangs me.

To men,
sex is the important bit, and foreplay is a waste of 30 minutes.

To women,
foreplay is the important bit, and sex is a waste of 30 seconds.

Her definition of a feminist...

A **strong, powerful** woman in control of her life, expertly juggling a home and career.

His definition of a feminist...

A **fat chick** who won't sleep with me. (And that's his definition of a lesbian, too.)

Dic**she**nary

Dicktionary

Condom
A healthy and mess-free item used for family planning and disease prevention.

A stupid piece of rubber with fiddly packaging that causes erection loss.

The pill
Birth-control method that causes nausea and weight gain and other unspeakable side effects, thus making intercourse unappealing.

A no-effort liberation from the tyranny of the condom.

Diaphragm
An unspeakably messy and impossible to insert cap of hell, usually found covered in dust.

A small trampoline for elves, sometimes covered in gross sticky stuff.

Foreplay
The fun, exciting, and good part of sex.

A multipartnered golf game, I think.

Vibrator
A good pal who always brings the orgasm home.

That little bastard thing that has made her grumpy with me ever since she bought it.

Threesome
Sex between a woman and two men.

Sex between a man and two women.

Foursome
A fun evening out with another nice couple.

Sex between a man and three women.

Dic**she**nary   **Dick**tionary

A family gathering
A pleasant time spent with one's closest relatives.

Sex with your woman and her three sisters.

Cunnilingus
A pleasant interlude on the journey to intercourse.

A tongue-numbing price to be paid for fellatio.

Fellatio
A mouth-numbing price to pay for jewelry.

God's gift to man.

Orgasm
An explosion of ecstasy caused by a vibrator.

An explosion of ecstasy caused by sex.

Anal sex
A practice illegal in many American states.

A practice apparently illegal in our bedroom.

Doggy style
A humiliating exposure of my big fat ass.

An exciting, animalistic sexual position.

Quickie
Every sexual encounter with your man.

A spontaneous and exciting sexual encounter with your woman.

Regular sex
At least once a week, often involving romance.

At least once a day, often involving a real woman.

Monogamy
Commitment to a relationship with one person.

Commitment to one person who doesn't know about any of the others yet.

Five reasons why she won't be having sex with you for the next six months:

1. You believed her when she said she didn't want you to do anything special for Valentine's Day.
2. You used her Jimmy Choos to hammer in a nail.
3. You told her you loved her big, sexy ass.
4. You mentioned that when she comes she sounds like two mountain goats fighting.
5. You told her you thought her best friend had lost weight.

Five good reasons you can give him so you won't have to have sex for six months:

1. My gynecologist said, blah blah blah... (he'll have stopped listening after the first three words).
2. I want to try for a baby.
3. What does green discharge mean?
4. I'm having an unusually long period.
5. We can have sex once for every time we have my mother to stay...

What **women** do to prepare for sex:

Wash, condition, shave, scrub, buff, pluck, clip, smooth, moisturize, powder, tone, coiffe, perfume, primp, stretch, trim, wax, conceal, highlight, tweeze, scrape, curl, straighten.

What **men** do to prepare for sex:
Get naked.

A couple are having a quiet evening at home. As they talk, a huge noise and bright, flashing lights seem to engulf the house, and then there is quiet, except for a strange, eerie hum coming from behind the house. Terrified, they grab a couple of golf clubs as weapons and creep out the back door of the house, where they see a **space ship** glowing menacingly at the bottom of their garden.

A door appears in the side of the ship and out step two aliens, one male, one female. The male alien says, "Do not be afraid, we come in peace to learn." So the human couple and the alien couple sit down and talk about their respective planets. Eventually, the **alien couple look at each other**, and the female alien says, "We are here for only one night. It would help us learn about you humans if we could mate with you."

The human husband and wife share a look and, realizing this is an opportunity few humans would ever get, they agree. They pair off, and the human woman takes the alien man to the bedroom. Fascinated, she watches as he takes off his silver uniform, but is disappointed to see that he is not well-endowed. "Oh, don't worry," he says, "all I have to do is this," at which he slaps himself across the forehead several times. Each time he slaps himself, **his penis grows one inch** in length. When she is satisfied with the length, she tells him that the girth is now too small, so he says, "No problem, all I have to do is this," and he starts pulling his ears, which makes the alien's penis grow in circumference.

After a night of unbelievable sex, they rejoin the others and the aliens leave. **"How was it for you?"** asks the woman's husband. "It was the most unbelievable experience of my life," she replies, "and what about you?"

"I hated it," he says.

"Why?" she asks.

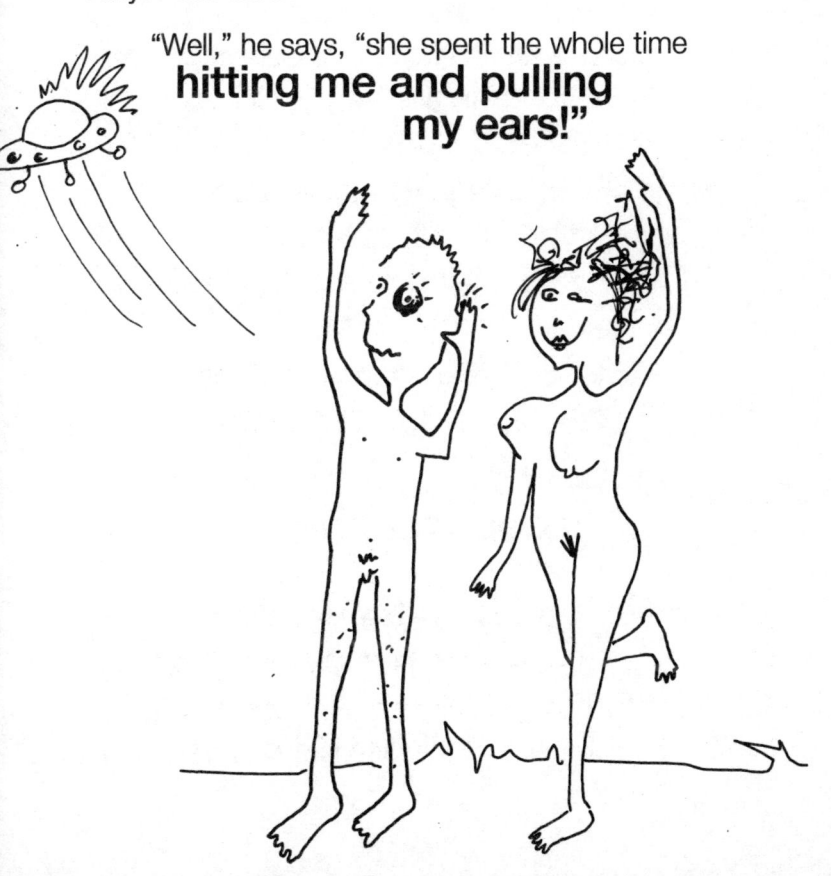

"Well," he says, "she spent the whole time **hitting me and pulling my ears!"**

Why do women like to be on top during sex?
So they can get off quickly afterwards to watch TV.

Why do men like to be underneath?
So they can fall asleep afterwards with the minimum of effort.

How do you know your relationship is doomed?
You look forward to the post-sex cigarette more than the sex itself.

Why shouldn't you have sex on the first date?
It embarrasses the restaurant staff.

How do you know your sex life is dead?
All you do when you sleep together is sleep together.

What do you do if he wants you to dress like a whore?
Charge him $50 an hour or $200 for the whole night.

Why is a penis like a puppy?

It's awake before you in the morning, always wants to be stroked, and sometimes you feel like having it neutered.

Why is it good to have a mirrored ceiling above the bed?

So you know when you're having sex with a vampire.

The erogenous zones on a woman:

Her breasts, her earlobes, her throat, the small of her back, her toes, her belly button, that little hollow in her throat, the back of her neck, her tummy (depending on whether she's feeling bloated or not), the soft skin on the inside of her thighs, her brain…

The erogenous zones on a man:

His cock.

Dicktionary

He says	**He means**
You're the sexiest woman in the world.	You're the sexiest woman in my bed.
I love you...	but only while we're having sex.
mmmngggrrffnn?	Is two minutes of oral sex enough for you?
This has never happened before.	**I'm borderline impotent.**
No, I like small breasts...	but SOME would be nice.
Oh, babe, you're the best.	... in your family anyway.
Did you come?	I wasn't aware of anything after your bra came off.
How was it for you?	Answer quick, I'll be asleep in ten seconds.
Oh God! Oh God!	Oh God! Please don't let me come yet! Football. Car engines. The square root of pi. Geometry. School. That film set in a school with **Michelle Pfeiffer**. **Michelle Pfeiffer**. No, not **Michelle Pfeiffer**! Too late! Oh God! **Unghhhhh.**

Dic**she**nary

She says	**She means**
Come on, take me now!	*ER* is on in ten minutes.
Oh, babe, you're the best!	When was the last time we painted the ceiling?
Grrnnffmmmrrrlt.	I think it's your turn to go down on me.
It's not size that counts.	Hey pal, you should carry a magnifying glass for that thing.
I think your aim is little off.	Get that thing out of my ass.
No, really, it's all right that I didn't come.	Hand me my vibrator and **shut the door behind you**.
A little to the left.	You can't even find the friggin' milk, how can I expect you to find my clitoris?
Oh God! Oh God!	I deserve **an Oscar** for this performance.

In a **man's** ideal world all **women** would:

1. Look like Carmen Electra.

2. Have **sex** like a Russian whore.

3. Know the rules of all sports and have a passionate interest in debating them.

4. And have good-looking charming friends that will act as his **sex slaves**.

In a **woman's** ideal world all **men** would:

1. After sex, turn into a pair of Manolo Blahniks.

2. Be interested in her **skincare** routine.

3. Build muscle tone from drinking beer.

4. And have good-looking, charming friends.

Jim the farmer went to market and bought 30 pigs for breeding. But being new to farming, he didn't know till he got them back to the farm that they were all female. So he called his neighbor, Farmer Bob, and asked if he could bring them over to mate with Farmer Bob's male pigs.

So, in the morning he brought them to Farmer Bob's and picked them up in the evening, saying to Farmer Bob, **"How will I know if they're pregnant?"** And Farmer Bob says, "Pigs don't normally graze. If they do, they're pregnant." The next morning, Farmer Jim gets up and sees that his pigs aren't grazing, so he brings his pigs back to Farmer Bob's farm and leaves them for another day with the male pigs.

The following morning, he says to his wife, "I can't bear to look, can you tell me if they're grazing?" So she looks out of the window and says, "No, they're not grazing, but they're all in the truck and one of them is **honking the horn.**"

CHAPTER THREE

Going Places Together

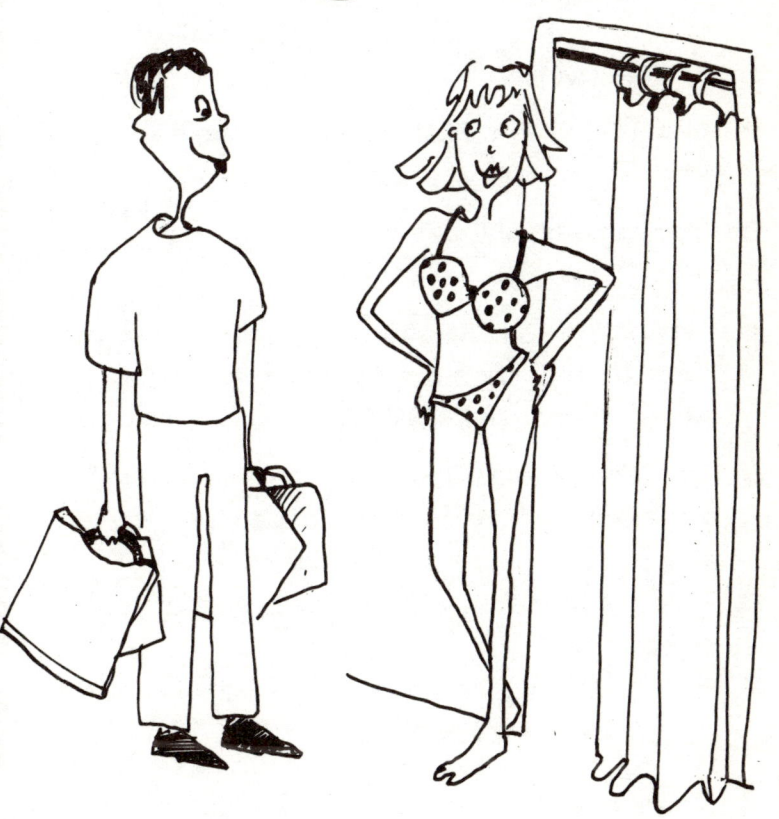

How to make the shopping experience more agreeable for a man:

There should be **play areas for men**, like there are for kids, in every shopping mall. You can drop your man off and pick him up later.

But here's what you can do in the **meantime**:

1. Promise to try on bikinis for at least ten minutes.

2. Keep **food treats** in your purse to be administered every 15 minutes.

3. Promise to be enthusiastic about plasma TVs with him.

4. To perk him up while shoe shopping, ask him to imagine which shoes you'd look best walking around the house **nude** in.

5. Don't bother to ask him what you look like in something—you're not going to pay any attention to what he says anyway.

6. Don't roll your eyes when he tells you that you look beautiful.

7. Promise to go to an action movie with him.

How to get your woman to go and see an action movie with you:

1. Tell her it's a tender romantic story about a woman experiencing a painful loss. But leave out the part about the 25-minute car chase and the high body count.

2. Tell her you're taking her out to dinner. (It's just that dinner will be a **hot dog and some popcorn**.)

3. On no account let slip that Vin Diesel is in it.

4. Appear surprised when she points out that she's the only woman in the movie theater.

5. Tell her it's a film about **marital** arts, then afterward pretend to be shocked that it was **martial** arts.

6. Promise to go shopping with her— as long as it's for bikinis or plasma TVs.

7. Tell her you are the man and you will decide what movies you see. (This may not work.)

A husband and wife are driving home after a party. After a while, the wife says to her husband, **"Darling, has anyone ever told you how sexy, good-looking, and fascinating you are to women?"**

The husband smiles, flattered, and says, **"Well, thank you, but no, they haven't."**

And the wife screams: **"So what the hell made you think that at the party tonight?"**

A man walks into a florist's and looks around him, confused. The assistant sees him and goes over to him. **"Can I help you?"** she asks.

"Yes," he replies, "I'd like to buy some flowers."

"Of course," she says, **"what have you got in mind?"**

The man looks confused again, and says, **"Well, I … I … I'm not really sure, I…"**

"Let me make it easier for you," she says. **"Why don't you tell me what you've done?"**

A man is at the Chanel counter buying expensive perfume for his wife.

"A surprise present for your wife?" asks the assistant.

"Certainly is," replies the man, "she's expecting a five-star trip to the Bahamas."

Her gym **fantasy**

I go to the gym to meet with my trainer. He tells me all the dieting and exercise has paid off and my body is **perfect**. He can do nothing else for me. I go on the step machine feeling strong and powerful. I can do anything. Everyone is staring at me because **I look so fabulous**. Supermodels are coming up to me asking my secret. Jennifer Lopez asks me how I got my perfect ass. And I can eat whatever I want and still look like this.

Her gym **reality**

Slog to the gym in the rain. What a stupid idea to walk instead of drive. Get hungry on way and buy a Snickers bar—hey, I'll burn it off. Arrive at door of gym doubled over with **exhaustion**.

Smiling receptionist says, "Good workout?"
"I just got here," I growl.

My trainer rolls his eyes in disgust as my chocolate from my Snickers bar is still on my face. I start walking on the treadmill; on either side of me everyone is running. I must look insane because I forgot my sports bra and I have to hold my breasts. Slip on a pool of my **own sweat** and my ass gets caught in the treadmill. Get carried downstairs past supermodels by three straining male trainers and placed in a taxi.

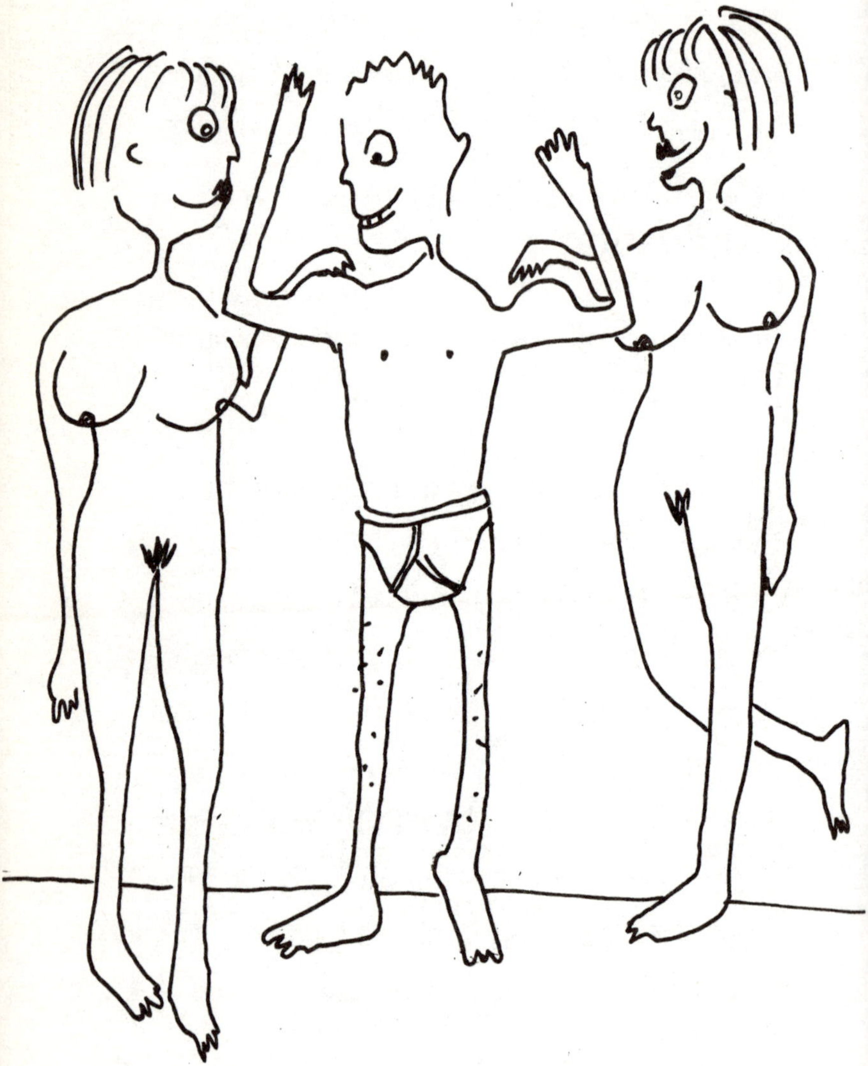

His gym fantasy

I'm just about to go into the shower when the door of the changing room opens and a beautiful blonde leans in and says, "Hi. The women's showers aren't working and the manager said that the team and I could use the men's showers. Do you mind?" I answer, "Sure." And I watch in amazement as ten more **stunning blondes** arrive giggling and talking, and start removing their clothes. We all go into the showers. "Ooh," someone says, "you've really been working out. Can we soap your big, bad muscles?" I stand there and **flex** as soap drips down my biceps. The first blonde says, "Have you ever made love with 11 women at once…?"

His gym reality

Must do something about scrawny arms. Go to bicep machine. Adjust weight from 300 pounds to a humiliating 50, while previous occupant sniggers and nudges fellow musclemen. Still have trouble pushing it. Feel like I'm back in school. Notice supermodel walking past. As she looks at me, I make extra effort. Feel something go in my back. I hear a shrill **scream of agony**. It's coming from me. Am carried downstairs by one female trainer and placed in taxi next to groaning plump woman. Our torn-up gym membership cards are thrown into the taxi after us by disgusted staff.

Reasons why men are better drivers

1. Better spatial awareness allows judgement of distances.

2. Unlikely to be distracted by sale dresses in windows of shops.

3. Men have never caused an accident by **checking lipstick** in the rearview mirror.

4. Men are less likely to think the life of a small furry animal crossing the road is more important than the lives of a car full of passengers.

5. Men are less likely to cry and be helpless if car breaks down.

6. Men are less likely to be running late and speeding because of six changes of outfit before setting off.

7. Men are more likely to have chosen car because of quality rather than "it's a **pretty color**."

8. Surely having a penis counts for something?

Reasons why **women** are better drivers

1. Fact: fewer accidents are caused by women.

2. Women are more likely to get you there, as men would rather have their penis cut off than ask for directions.

3. More likely to be watching the road instead of honking to make girls turn around.

4. Women don't think it's an affront to their femininity if passengers point out they are driving on the wrong side of the road.

5. Women's **multitasking skills** enable them to drink coffee and drive with no danger to passengers.

6. Women are less likely to enter a **pointless race** with a bozo who overtakes them.

7. No accident has ever been caused by a male passenger giving oral sex to a female driver.

8. Less likely than men to wrap the car around a tree while trying to recreate a drag race from *The Fast and the Furious* in the middle of town.

A woman is stopped by a police officer for speeding. The officer walks over to the car and notices a number of dangerous **long knives** on the back seat.

Alarmed, he asks the woman what they're for. "Oh, those," she laughs, "they're **machetes**. I'm a juggler, and they're part of my act." "Well, show me," he says, and she does. She gets out of the car and starts to **juggle** first two, then three, and eventually seven machetes, in an amazing display.

Just then, a couple drive by in another car, arguing. The wife looks at the juggling and says to her husband, "You're never driving after a drink again.

Look at the test they're giving now!"

A man is speeding down a narrow country road at night. Suddenly, another car appears around a corner in front of him and swerves, only just missing him.

The woman leans out of her window and shouts, **"Pig!"**

The man leans out his window and shouts, **"Bitch!"**

The man sets off again. As he rounds the next corner, he crashes into a **pig** in the middle of the road.

Car parking instructions

For men:

1. Find a space.
2. Reverse in.

For women:

1. Find a space.
2. Realize it's probably **too small**, given that it doesn't have two empty parking spaces on either side of it.
3. Ignore **man** trying to guide you into space because he doesn't think you can park.
4. While being angry about this, ruefully accept that he may have a point.
5. Back out slowly, **almost hitting** oncoming car.
6. Drive around for half an hour running out of gas.
7. Finally, notice five empty disabled parking spaces. Take one and limp into shopping mall.

A man phones his **new girlfriend** and says, "Look, I'm really sorry, but my car is broken down."

"Don't worry," she says, "I'll come and pick you up."

When she arrives, he notices her car is painted red on one side and blue on the other. He walks round the car twice and says: **"Your car—why is it painted red on one side and blue on the other?"**

"Oh," she replies, "that's for when I get into accidents. You should hear the witnesses contradicting each other!"

CHAPTER FOUR

Tying the Knot

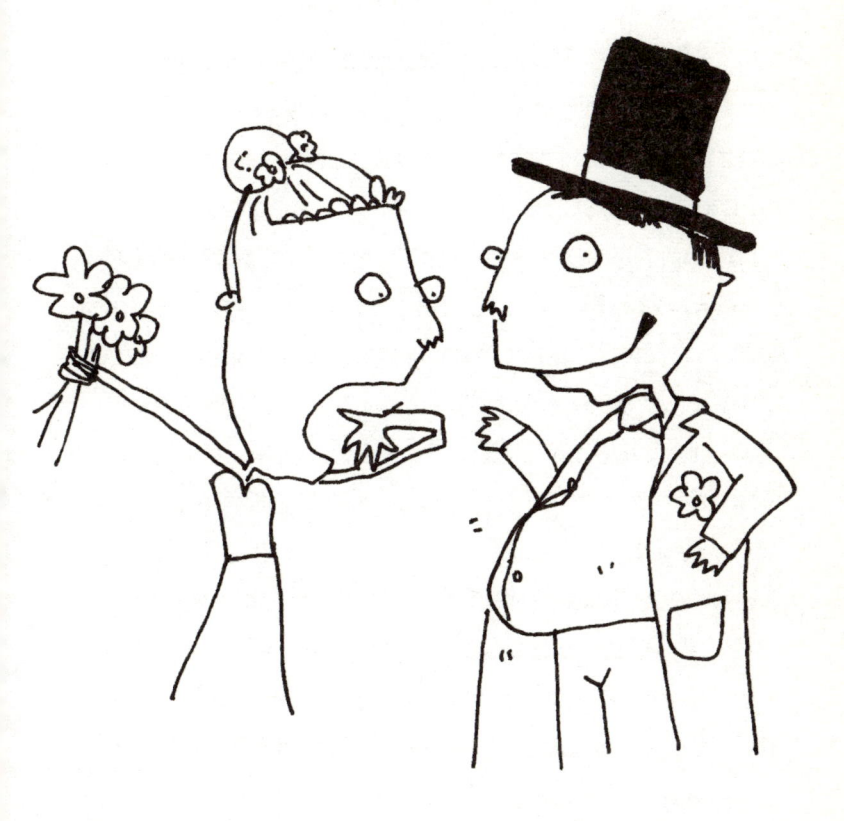

He says:
Why buy the cow when the milk is free?

She says:
It is not worth buying the pig for the six measly ounces of sausage.

Mike's having terrible trouble.

He loves his parents and wants to please them, but his mother continually disapproves of the women he brings home to meet them. Finally, he thinks he's found the **perfect woman**: she looks like his mother, she sounds like his mother—she has all the same attitudes as his mother. He brings her around to his parents for dinner, and she gets on incredibly well with his mother, and they chat and laugh together all evening. The next day, Mike phones his mother and says, "Well, what did you think of Mary?" And his mother says, "I think she's wonderful, but, there's a problem." "What," asks Mike, "is the problem now?" "Well," replies his mother, **"your father can't stand her."**

What to say when you meet the parents

for her:

What to say:	Mm, what a delicious dinner, Mrs. Smith.
What not to say:	No wonder he has the palette of a peasant!
What to say:	Your house is in perfect order, Mrs. Smith.
What not to say:	I've seen homeless people with cleaner cardboard boxes!
What to say:	Oh I'd love to see all the home movies.
What not to say:	... But I have to commit suicide now.

for him:

What to say:	I love your sofa.
What not to say:	I can't wait to bang your daughter on this sofa.
What to say:	You have a great-looking family.
What not to say:	I'll be knocking up your daughters one by one.
What to say:	Susan tells me you're planning an around-the-world cruise.
What not to say:	Are you, like, spending our inheritance?

Family survival guide for **her:**

When his parents keep mentioning how perfect his **last girlfriend** was, remind them what a pity it was that a jury didn't agree.

When his parents point out your humble origins, inform them of their son's **humble skills** in bed.

When there are too many family members for you to remember, **fantasize** about which ones you would execute.

When his parents try to convert you to their religion, tell them that their son has agreed to convert to yours: **devil worship**.

When his father drunkenly caresses your thigh under the table, remove your bra and loudly ask, "Hey, you want to grab these, too?"

Family survival guide for **him:**

When her parents insist on you sleeping in separate bedrooms, inform them that the same arrangement will apply to them when they visit you.

When her parents insist they want a big, traditional wedding for their daughter, tell them you want a big, **traditional dowry**.

When her parents show concern about your ability to support their daughter, tell them your prostitution ring is beginning to show profits.

When her parents start hinting about grandchildren, inquire as to whether your **illegitimate children** count.

When her father brags about his aristocratic ancestry, smile and reminisce about your upbringing among banjo-playing Appalachian mountain folk.

The advice column

> DEAR ADVICE COLUMN,
>
> MY GIRLFRIEND AND I ARE GETTING MARRIED SOON. SHE HAS GONE INSANE PLANNING THE WEDDING. SHE HAS BECOME COMPLETELY CONTROLLING AND I DON'T GET A SAY IN ANYTHING. WHAT SHOULD I DO?
>
> SIGNED HAPLESS FIANCÉ

Dear Hapless Fiancé,

Your girlfriend has been dreaming of her wedding her whole life. She saw herself looking beautiful, in the perfect dress, with everyone telling her how wonderful she was. She has not been dreaming of you. Sorry to tell you, but you are unimportant and superfluous. You could put anyone in a suit and she would still have her perfect time. Hope you enjoy her big day.

> Dear Advice Column,
>
> I'm getting married soon and my boyfriend is insisting on having a say in some of the planning. He even wants to have a vegetarian choice for dinner, as some people in his family don't eat meat. He's ruining everything. What should I do?
>
> Signed Pretty Bride

Dear Pretty Bride,

How very selfish of him. Who cares what his family eats. Are they paying for the wedding? We didn't think so. Just ignore him. What does he know? He's just a guy.

Advantages to being married

For her:

A wedding ring will make your single friends jealous, even if they're prettier or skinnier than you.

You never have to swallow again.

His *casa* is your *casa*.

If you should "accidentally" kill him, you'll get all his money.

You have a New Year's Eve date for life.

You get to choose unflattering bridesmaids' dresses for your best friends.

You can finally give his mother the finger and there's nothing she can do about it.

It will make your **other boyfriend** really jealous.

For him:

Ummm...
At least she'll stop nagging you to marry her...

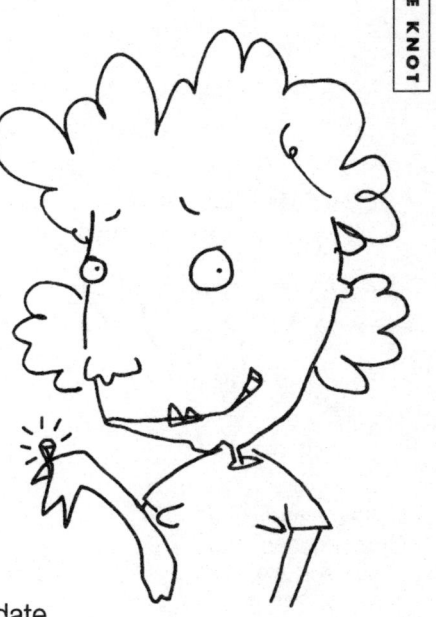

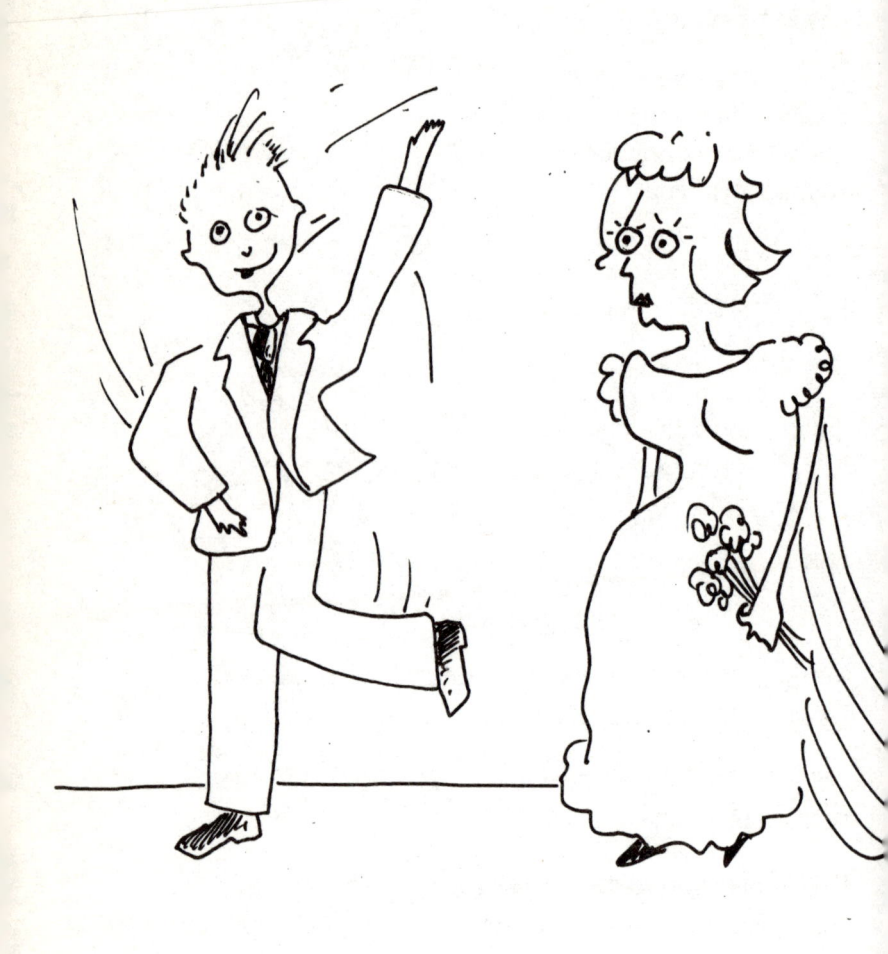

Advantages to not marrying your woman

Keep dangling the promise of a wedding ring and you can get her to do anything.

She has **no legal claim** to your *Star Wars* figurine collection.

The pleasure of watching her becoming angry and embittered as all her friends get married.

You won't wake up naked and **chained** to a lamppost the morning after your **bachelor** party.

You won't have to suffer her stepbrother following you around the reception, winking at you and telling you she's "quite a girl."

You can take all the money you've saved up for her **engagement ring** and buy a Harley Davidson.

No wedding reception = **No one to see what a crap dancer you are.**

On their honeymoon night, the burly groom took off his pants and asked his bride to put them on.

The waist alone was twice her body. She said, **"I can't wear your pants."**

"That's right," intoned the groom, "And don't you forget it. I'm the one who wears the pants in this family."

The bride took off her panties and asked her husband to try them on. "No way. I can't get into your pants."

"That's right. And that's the way it will be until you change your attitude."

"How would you feel about being wife number three?"
"Why, are you divorced?"
"No, I'm a Mormon."

What's the similarity between toilets and wedding anniversaries?
Men always miss both of them.

Tom and Mary arrive at the reception on their wedding day.

They are both really excited, having just got married, and Mary beckons Tom into a quiet room and locks the door. Sometime later, they both emerge.

Tom's best man calls him over and says, "Hey, you look so happy! What happened?"

Tom beams and says,
"I just got my best blowjob ever!"

Meanwhile Mary's bridesmaid says to her:
"You look so happy! What happened?"

Mary says,
"I just gave my last blowjob ever!"

Things not to say on your wedding night

Him:

Oh ... now you've got the veil off ... I thought I was marrying your sister.

The video guys are here because I want to record every part of our wedding day.

Let's get this over with quick 'cos **the game starts in five minutes**.

Now, before we have sex, you'd better fold my clothes and clean the house.

Tomorrow I'll introduce you to my other wives.

I thought it would be fun if Cindy the waitress joined us for a threesome.

Is it OK if all my drinking friends watch?

Ooh, I've been dying to try on your wedding dress all day!

My parents are waiting outside to show off the bloodstained sheets.

Now, which suitcase did I pack the **whips and chains in**?

Her:

Where's the bottle? I've never had sex sober before.

You know I told you I didn't want to have sex before our wedding night ... well, that was because my doctor told me I needed to wait six months for the chlamydia to clear up.

Wait a minute, I've just got to take this call from my ex-boyfriend.

I've got you some literature about penile implant surgery.

Him? Oh, he's the Rabbi. He's going to **circumcise you** before we go any further.

Is this a good time to mention my heroin addiction?

Let's make this night last. My five-year jail sentence starts tomorrow.

Just place $200 on the bedside table or you're getting nothing, pal.

Well, sweetie, my debts are now our debts, and there's a man named Vinnie waiting outside to see you…

Oooh! Sorry, but that **sex-change surgery** is still a little painful.

Jim and Tina have just got married
and, to save money, they spend their wedding night at the bride's parents' house.

Unfortunately, their bedroom is right next to Tina's parents' bedroom, and as they start to make love, the bedsprings squeak. Realizing they're going to have to go to a hotel anyway, they quietly start to pack a suitcase, but find they've overpacked it, and it won't close.

Tina's father is lying awake next door and hears Tina say, **"Let me sit on it."** A few moments later, he hears Jim say, **"Let's both sit on it."**

Tina's dad rushes for the bedroom door, saying to his wife,

"This, I've got to see!"

A woman is sitting alone at a bar.

A **drunken man** comes in, walks over to her, puts his hand up her blouse, and starts fondling her breasts.

She jumps up and slaps him in the face.

Horrified, he stops and apologizes. **"I'm really sorry! It's just that you look exactly like my wife."**

"You stupid, drunk, useless piece of shit!" she screams.

"Amazing," he says. **"You sound just like her too!"**

CHAPTER FIVE

Domestic Bliss

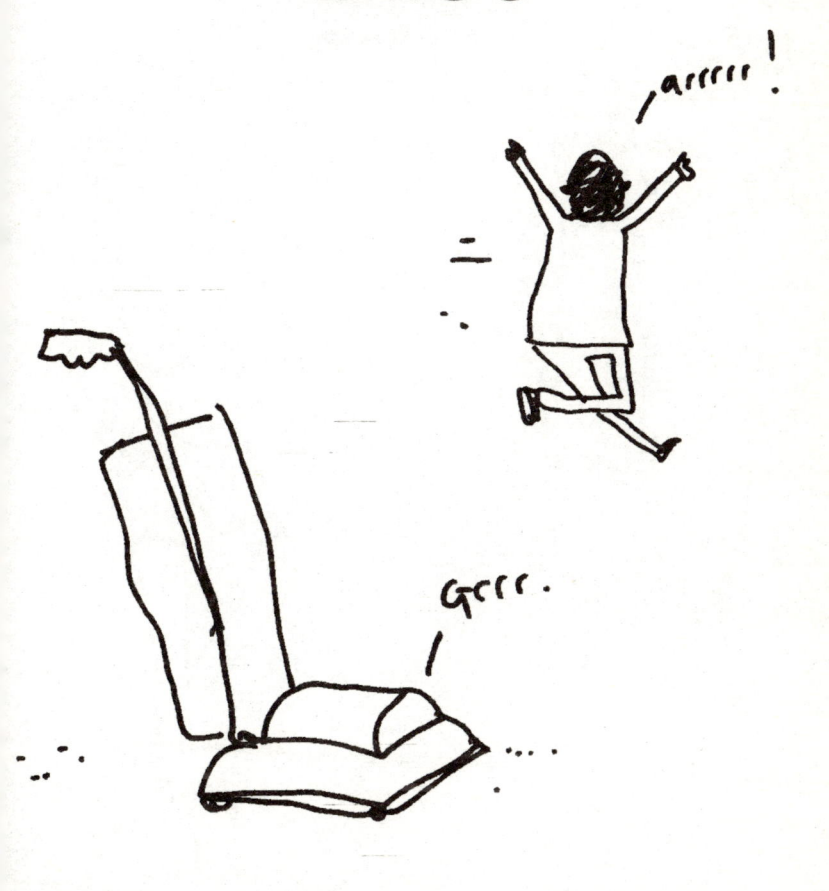

80 • ADAM VS. EVE

What **she** wants to wear around the house:

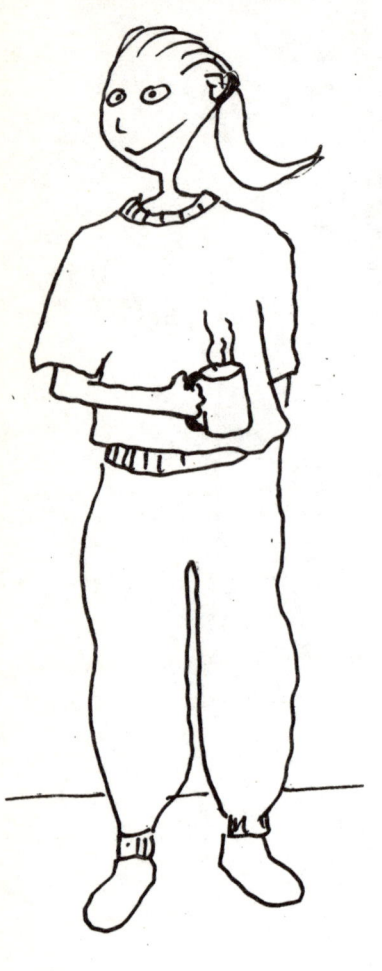

What **he** wants her to wear around the house:

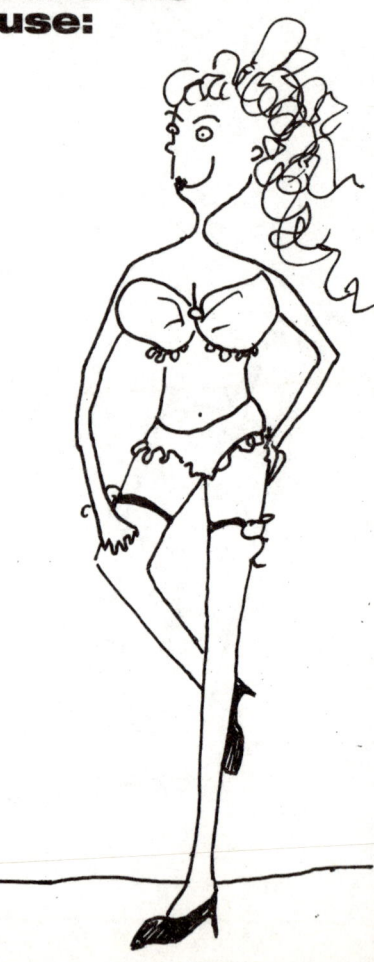

What **he** wants to wear around the house:

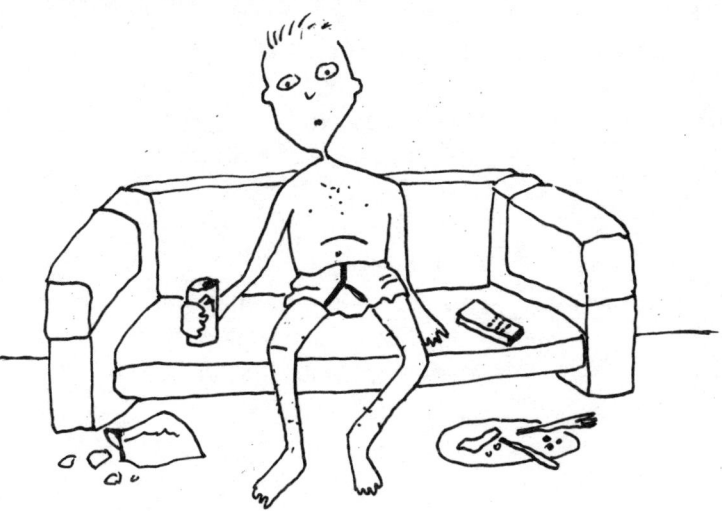

What **she** wants him to wear around the house:

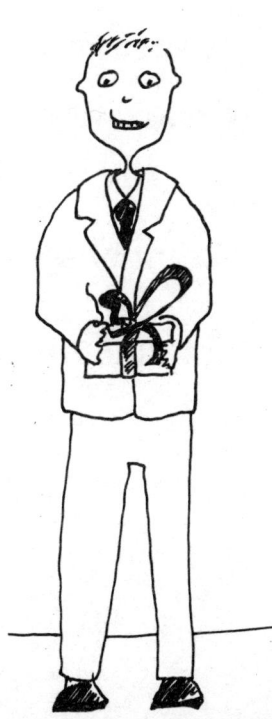

He says... she says...

What he says: I'll never be as good a cook as you.

What he means: One more burnt steak and I'll never have to cook again.

What she says: You don't do your share of the housework.

What she means: I am an insane **clean freak**, who should be cleaning the floors in a lunatic asylum with my toothbrush.

What he says: You don't look after me enough.

What he means: You don't look after me as much as my mother thinks you should.

What she says: You don't look after me enough.

What she means: I should have married someone richer.

What he says:	Let's go out to dinner tonight.
What he means:	I can see the anger in your eyes and the carving knife in your hand.
What she says:	Let's go out to dinner tonight.
What she means:	If I have to cook another dinner it'll be your liver we're eating!

What she says:	Will you look at fabric swatches with me?
What she means:	Obviously I don't care about your opinion, but I know you like to be involved.
What he says:	Yes, I'll look at fabric swatches with you.
What he means:	Kill me, **kill me now!**

What she says:	We need to repaint the whole house.
What she means:	You will never relax on a weekend ever again!
What he says:	Sure, I'll repaint the house.
What he means:	We both know I'm not going to repaint the house.

What she says: We need to buy a new bed.
What she means: If I can't change my husband, **I'm damn well changing something!**

What he says: Sure, let's buy a new bed.
What he means: Oh goody, a new place to do it!

What she says: I've paid the phone bill.
What she means: He'll never find out how often I talk to my best friend in Paris.

What he says: I've paid the phone bill.
What he means: She'll never find out how often I talk to **my mistress in L.A.**

What she says: I've ironed your shirts.
What she means: I love you and care for you. I am willing to undertake this dreary task to show my love for my man. I am truly the most perfect and wonderful wife who ever lived. Please get down on your knees and worship me. I am woman, **hear me roar!**

What he says: Thank you for ironing my shirts.
What he means: What was your name again?

What she says: I don't believe in sex **before** marriage.
What she means: I don't believe in sex **after** marriage either.

What he says: I don't want you to rush into anything you're not ready for…
What he means: **NEXT!!!!!!!!**

Domestic instructions for **men** and **women**:

How do you know when the dinner is cooked?

Her answer: When the delicious aroma of food is wafting around the kitchen.
His answer: When the smoke alarm goes off (that's also how you know the ironing is done).

How do you know when it's time to clean?

Her answer: When your neat feminine order is slightly disturbed.
His answer: You don't remember having bought a carpet made of beer cans.

When should you wash clothes?

Her answer: Saturday mornings for whites, Tuesday evenings for colors.
His answer: When tramps start giving you money.

How often should you wash the sheets?

Her answer: Once a week, whether they need it or not.
His answer: Once a year, whether they need it or not.

When should you throw out old food?

Her answer: When the best-before date is up.
His answer: When scientists are exploring your refrigerator for new forms of Penicillin.

When should you buy Christmas presents?

Her answer: In the January sales after the previous Christmas.
His answer: One minute to midnight on December 24th, at the gas station—just after mailing Christmas cards.

The advice column

DEAR ADVICE COLUMN,

MY GIRLFRIEND WANTS ME TO MOVE IN WITH HER, BUT HER HOUSE IS SO NEAT AND PRISTINE, AND SHE WON'T LET ME HAVE ANY OF MY GUY STUFF AROUND. WHAT SHOULD I DO?

SIGNED SLOPPY BUT IN LOVE

Dear Sloppy,
First of all, don't worry about your mess, women love picking up after men. Nothing thrills them more than collecting our dirty socks and underwear and putting them in the laundry basket. It makes them feel feminine. And needed.

Second, is your parents' house full of guy stuff? Your grandparents'? Any house of any couple you've ever been to in your entire life? Wake up and smell the coffee! Once you are with a woman, your say in decorating is over.

Dear Advice Column,

I want my boyfriend to move in with me, but he's messy and has all kinds of cheap, stupid stuff he wants to put in my nice house. What should I do?

Signed Pretty House

Dear Pretty House,
Don't worry about the mess. Men are so easily trained. They love being told what to do, and they feel so masculine being nagged to pick up their dirty clothes.

As for his stuff, he will be grateful to you if you throw it all out. Do it when he isn't home. How you both will laugh when he finds out the drinking mug he bought in New Orleans when he was 16 is gone forever. And do get rid of his bedside lamp shaped like a football. It will be a bonding experience.

Dic**she**nary

Clean
Clean or germ-free.

Dish-washing
Cleansing dishes after a meal.

Changing the sheets
Removing the dirty sheets and replacing them with clean, fresh ones.

Ironing
Removing creases from loved ones' apparel for maximum smartness.

Laundry basket
A convenient repository for the containment of dirty clothes en route for the washing machine.

Floor
A wooded or carpeted area that must be constantly kept clean.

Dicktionary

Not actually suppurating with typhoid germs.

Putting dishes into the sink and hoping they magically clean themselves (by the same house fairy that also irons).

Buying new ones every five years once the old ones turn black.

An ancient process not needed since the invention of new shirts.

A place to find underwear and socks to wear.

A place to keep dirty clothes and towels.

Dic**she**nary

Vacuuming
Dull but necessary activity needed to clean the floor.

Dust
The accumulated dirt that needs to be periodically removed from surfaces.

Bed
A place of refuge and rest after a hard day, and for gentle, amorous bonding.

Dicktionary

A noisy disturbance while watching football.

The cool stuff you can write your name in.

A place to fuck, fart, and fall asleep.

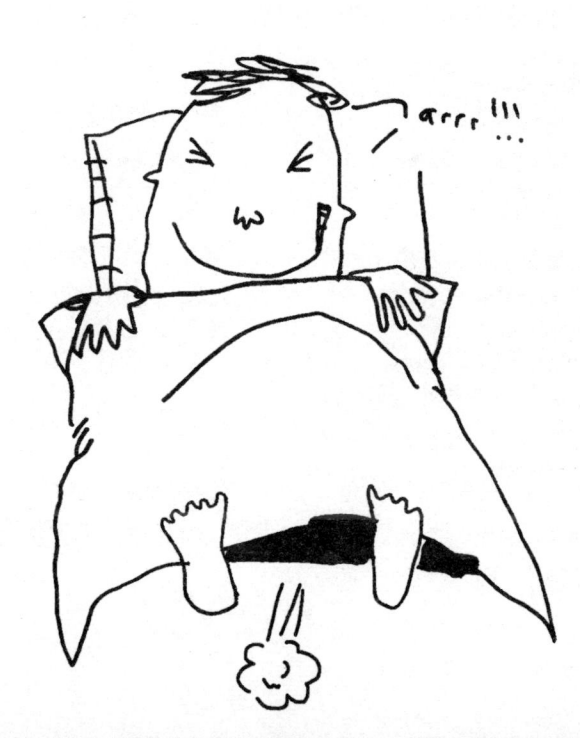

Her shopping list:

Fresh vegetables	Extra Virgin olive oil
Fruits	Wholewheat bread
Herbs	24 pack of Diet Cokes
Rice cakes	Lean Cuisine meals for one
Cottage cheese	Tampons
Skim milk	Giant chocolate cake
Soy milk	
Cranberry juice	

His shopping list:

KETCHUP	MONTH'S SUPPLY
24 PACK OF BEERS	OF PORN MAGS
PRINGLES	MORE KETCHUP
BAKED BEANS	BARBECUE SAUCE
CHEESE SLICES	~~CLEANING SUPPLIES AND~~
PIZZAS	~~AIR FRESHENER~~
SLICED WHITE BREAD	
MONTH'S SUPPLY OF FROZEN TV DINNERS	

An efficiency expert is coming toward the end of his lecture. "Many of these principles are highly effective in the workplace. However, I recommend that you do not try them in the home."

"Why not?" calls a man from the audience.

"Well," replies the expert, **"I spent many years observing my wife's breakfast routine.** She would move between the refrigerator, the oven, the kitchen cabinets, and the table, usually carrying only one item at a time. Finally, I said to her, "It would be far more efficient if you were to plan your journeys and carry several items at a time."

"Did it save time?" asks the man in the audience.

"Well, it did," replies the expert. **"Breakfast used to take her 25 minutes to prepare. Now, it takes me only seven."**

A woman is at her wits' end. **Her husband never does anything around the house** to help his busy wife, claiming that it's women's work. But one day she comes home to find the house immaculately tidy, all the vacuuming and laundry done, the ironing neatly folded, and dinner waiting for her on a beautifully laid table. Astonished, she asks her husband what is happening. He tells her he's just read a magazine article pointing out that a working wife is much more likely to want **to make love** if she is not having to do all the housework.

Next day, she tells her best friend all about it. **"So what happened?"** her friend asks.

"It was amazing," she said. "The dinner was superb, he then washed the dishes, he put away the ironing, helped the kids do their homework, and then tucked them up in bed."

"But what about afterwards?" asks the friend.

"Nothing happened," she replied. **"He was too tired from all the housework."**

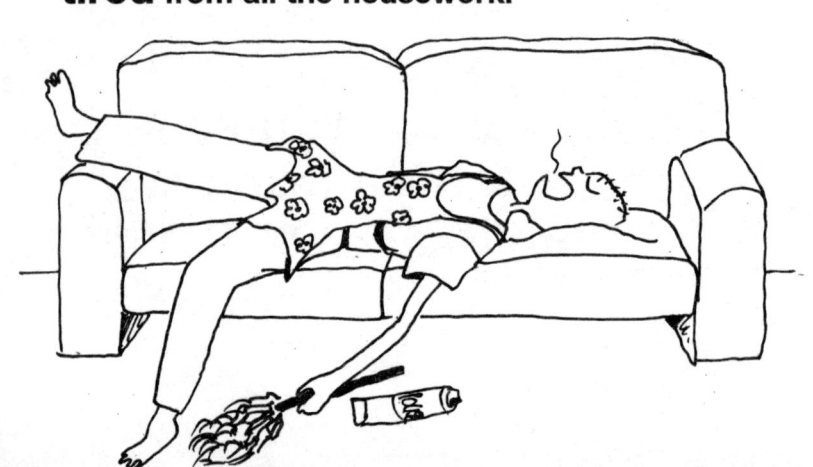

How do get your man to vacuum?
Point out that a vacuum cleaner is a "gadget."

How do you get your woman to stop nagging you to vacuum?
Tell her tests show vacuuming has been proven to burn 1,000 calories a minute.

How do you get your man to repair the cracks in the bedroom ceiling?
Point out that it means there'll be nothing to distract you when you're having sex.

How do you get your woman to stop obsessing about the cleanliness of the oven?
Just clean it once, for God's sake!

Is it true that the way to a man's heart is through his stomach?
Yes, although you have to aim the knife upward.

How do you avoid forgetting your wife's birthday?
Forget it once—you're guaranteed never to forget it again.

CHAPTER SIX

Advice for the Sexes

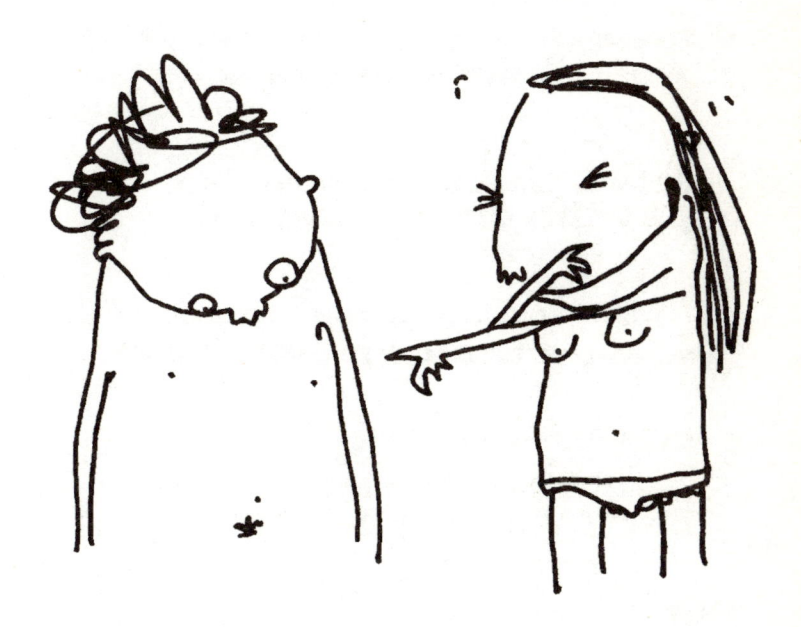

Words of wisdom

Women think they can take the man they met and improve him. What they don't realize is that the man they met was **the best he'll ever be**, because he was hiding all his faults from her and will spend the rest of his life slipping back into them.

Men want their women to stay exactly the same.

Men want to marry their mothers: then they can continue to **behave like children**.

Women want to marry their fathers: that way someone else will always **pay the credit card bill**.

Men want to put their woman on a pedestal: that way, they can **look up her skirt**.

Women want men to put them on a pedestal, look up their skirts, and give them head until the day they die.

Women are the only members of the household who know how to decorate a home.

A man's idea of **home improvement** is to badly hammer nails, and buy either navy blue or brown sheets.

If it's got **tires or testicles**, you're going to have trouble with it.

If it's got **breasts and lip gloss**, you're going to spend a lot of time saying, "You're so right and I'm so wrong."

A **man's libido** is like a martini: Anytime, anyplace, and anywhere.

A **woman's libido** is like champagne: Fiddly, difficult to uncork, and only available on special occasions.

A **woman** can look after her man through flu, pregnancy, and death.

A **man** falls apart at the first sign of a cold.

Don't ever learn how to iron, otherwise you will spend the rest of your life doing it.

Don't ever learn how to **put up shelves**; you'll end up doing it for everyone she has ever met.

He'll love your friends and want to have sex with at least three of them.

She'll hate your friends and want you to ditch at least three of them.

Every **man** wants to have sex with two women. So does every woman, but that's so she'll have someone to talk to afterward.

Women would make their lives so much easier if they would stop asking men what they're thinking about. He's thinking about **food, sex, or football**. Now move on!

Men never wonder what women are thinking about. But in case you're wondering, they are thinking about why you're **so quiet**.

No matter what **she says**, she wishes you made more money.

No matter what he says, he wishes you had **bigger boobs**.

Even if you look exactly like Brad Pitt, **she** still fantasizes about doing it with Brad Pitt.

Even if you look exactly like Catherine Zeta Jones, he still **fantasizes** about doing it with Pamela Anderson.

Women leave a relationship when they can't stand it another minute.

Men leave when they find someone better.

As they get older, women **get crazier**.

And men **stop talking**.

A **woman** shows how much she loves her man by carefully washing and ironing his shirts.

A **man** shows how much he loves his woman by leaving the room to fart.

Or, at least, leaving the sofa...

When getting married, choosing **the right man** is less important than choosing the right dress. After all, a wedding photo is for life.

Choose **your wife** carefully. After all, this is the face you'll be looking at in the divorce court.

The advice column

DEAR ADVICE COLUMN,

I AM MEETING MY GIRLFRIEND'S PARENTS FOR THE FIRST TIME. HOW DO I GET THEM TO LIKE ME?

SIGNED, EAGER AND IN LOVE.

Dear Eager and In Love,

Unless you are a convicted serial killer or a wanted terrorist, they will love you. They have been waiting for someone to come and take their daughter off their hands for a long time, and quite frankly, they'd given up hope. Even if you set their house on fire, they'd still like you.

Dear Advice Column,

My boyfriend is taking me to meet his parents this weekend. I believe he has mentioned to them that he wants to marry me. What kind of reception can I expect?

Signed Engaged and In Love.

Dear Engaged and In Love,

First of all, you're not good enough for him. Do you know how many single women there are out there? All the girlfriends he had before you were terrific. They were so pretty and seemed like they would be good homemakers. Plus, they had successful careers, which they would be willing to give up like a shot. Your fiancé is quite a catch. Plus, we understand that his childhood sweetheart is in town for the weekend, too. If you're not already crying, then you may, just may, be strong enough to handle this weekend.

Etiquette for modern men

A thank you note is not expected after oral sex, **but grunting, farting, and falling asleep are not appreciated.**

Always holding the door open for her is good. **Holding the door open for her when she's leaving you for good is not necessary.**

You only have to thank her mother for dinner. **You do not, despite how much she asks, have to have sex with her.**

While it is good to make friends with her female friends, it is not a good idea to make passes at them. **However, if one of her friends makes a pass at you, it is impolite to refuse. Or, at least, that's what you can tell your girlfriend later.**

If you meet a woman speed dating, she will not appreciate it later if you practice speed coming.

Buy flowers for her at every opportunity. **That way, she will not be suspicious when you buy them out of guilt for having slept with someone else.**

She will not appreciate it if you point at her sister and say, **"Hey, I bet she goes like a rabbit!"**

Never shout your lover's name when you're in bed together. **Especially if you're with your wife at the time.**

After performing oral sex it is not polite to spit and say, **"Yikes! I'm never doing that again."**

Etiquette for modern women

It is not appropriate to clone his credit card and embark on **spending sprees**.

Turning up late on occasion is tolerable.
Turning up late, drunk, and smelling of cum is not!

Sexy nude dancing in front of the TV during a football game will only lead to resentment at the choice he is being forced to make. **And you may not like the choice he makes.**

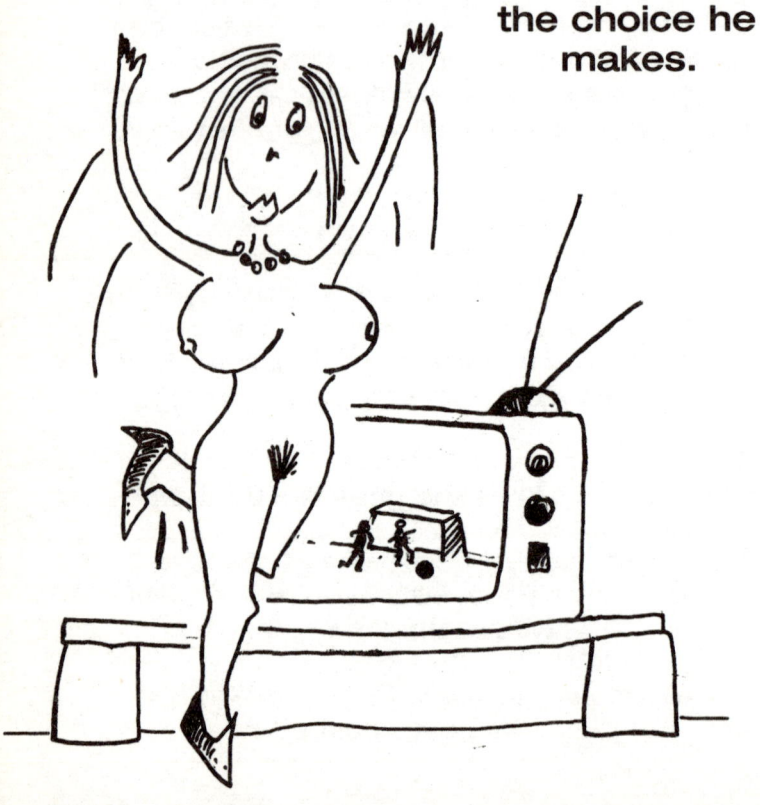

You only have to thank his mother for cooking dinner. **It is not necessary to thank her for bringing this wonderful man into the world.**

It is not considered top drawer to post pictures of his **small penis on the internet.**

It is impolite and self-defeating to denigrate his previous girlfriends. **Remember, the same man who chose them, chose you.**

If you find his secret stash of porn, do not wave it in his face and call him a pervert. **Instead, discreetly slip a sexy nude picture of yourself into one of them.**

Do not have your man's name tattooed on you. You will be faced with expensive laser surgery, or **having to go out with men with that name for the rest of your life**.

Insisting he wears a condom is fine. **However, it is thoughtless to insist he wears ten because his penis isn't big enough!**

After you've finished performing oral sex, **it is not polite to bring in a team of dental hygienists to detoxify your mouth.**

Reasons why it's great to be a **man**:

1. No one makes remarks when you hit **35** and you're still not married.
2. There isn't a half-hour wait to use the bathroom.
3. You can wear the same clothes day after day and no one notices.
4. You can **pee anywhere**—and are encouraged to do so.
5. No matter how **bad** the sex is, you still have an orgasm.
6. No one tells you look tired if you're not wearing make-up.
7. Looking at thin, beautiful women doesn't depress you.
8. You can be **ugly** and still be considered a great catch.
9. You can have a great time slumping on the couch, watching football and scratching yourself.
10. Your **penis** is a constant source of entertainment.

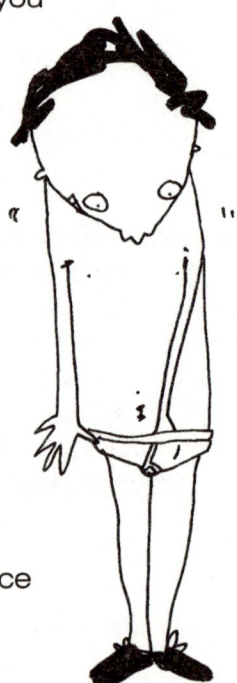

Reasons why it's great to be a **woman:**

1. You don't have to find **taxis** in the rain.
2. Shoe shopping is a blissful joy you can't put into words.
3. Once you have a partner, you never have to carry a suitcase again.
4. **Lip gloss** is a constant source of entertainment.
5. You can pretty much get out of doing anything just by saying "cramps."
6. The thrill of the perfect manicure.
7. You can cry and still **look sexy**.
8. You get to be the one who asks, in the middle of the night, "Did you hear something?" and stay comfortably in bed, while he has to sleepily stumble around in the dark.
9. You can be a feminist and still have him pay for everything.
10. You get to wear the engagement ring.

Reasons why it sucks to be a **man**:

1. Even though it's her period you still have to go out and buy tampons in the middle of the night.
2. You have to kill all the insects—**even the big, scary ones**.
3. You have to give her your jacket when it's cold—and then **listen to her complain** that it spoils her outfit.
4. A woman will never know the misery of going bald—unless she's a Russian shotputter.
5. She eats all your fries because apparently the calories don't count if she didn't order them herself.
6. You get blamed for **the bad behavior** of all the men in the world, including Saddam Hussein and all her previous boyfriends.
7. **You'll never know the pleasure of wearing a beautiful, floaty chiffon dress—outside of her bedroom, anyway.**
8. One word: IKEA.

Reasons why it sucks to be a **woman:**

1. Having your bikini line waxed.

2. Waiting for him to call.

3. Wasting your entire life thinking you're too fat.

4. The moment you realize no one is ever going to discover your potential to be a supermodel.

5. Sooner or later, no matter how long you put it off, you'll have to give him **a blowjob**.

6. They have yet to invent really cute high-heeled hiking shoes.

7. Being considered a slut just because you banged the whole football team.

8. You'll never get your hands on the TV remote.

What he says... what she hears...

I'm not looking for a serious relationship.	Go and choose yourself a wedding dress.
I'd like children someday...	You should stop taking the pill.
I love your figure.	You're too fat.
Go on, have dessert.	I want you to get fat so that no other man will find you attractive and you'll be trapped, trapped, do you hear me?!
I love you.	I want to have sex.

What she says... what he hears...

I'd like a cuddle.	I want to have sex.
You look good in that shirt.	I want to have sex.
I'm cooking Italian tonight.	I want to eat, then I want to have sex.
I don't want to have sex.	I don't want to have sex this minute, but if you keep pestering me, I will.
No, I really don't want to have sex.	I want to give you a blowjob.

If a **man** were a woman for a day he would:

Play with **his breasts** for hours.

Try to get off with a lesbian.

Go to communal changing rooms.

See whether he'd be **whistled at** by construction workers.

Read *Cosmopolitan* to see if it actually made sense now.

Have **sex with lots of people** and enjoy being called a slut.

If a **woman** were a man for a day she would:

Walk past a construction site to enjoy not being harassed.

Go to a bar to enjoy **not being harassed**.

Go to work and get promoted.

Walk alone at night feeling safe and secure.

Eat whatever she damn well pleased.

Feel the **thrill** of walking in comfortable shoes.

Look on the bright side of...

Finding his pubic hairs on the soap: At least he's washing the damned thing...

Premature ejaculation: At least it shows how much he fancies you...

His horrible snoring: At least he's at home in bed.

Him leaving the toilet seat up: At least he's not peeing all over the seat.

Him remaining silent all the time: At least he's not boring you with all his tedious crap.

He tracks mud into the house: At least he's still coming home.

He forgets your birthday: At least he doesn't remember you're a year older.

He's having an affair with your neighbor: At least somebody else finds him attractive.

He's leaving you for someone else: At least your soap will stay pube-free.

Look on the bright side of...

Her nagging you: Erm...

Her finding excuses not to have sex: Well...

You having to do all the heavy shit around the house:
There must be some bright side...

Her spending all your hard-earned money on pillows:
Yeah, what's the deal with that?

Having her mother to stay: Enough, already!

Her making you take the dog out in the rain: Well, that's not so bad, he's my only real friend...

Spending hours waiting while she tries on outfits:
OK, that's it! I'm gone!

CHAPTER SEVEN

Diary of a Relationship

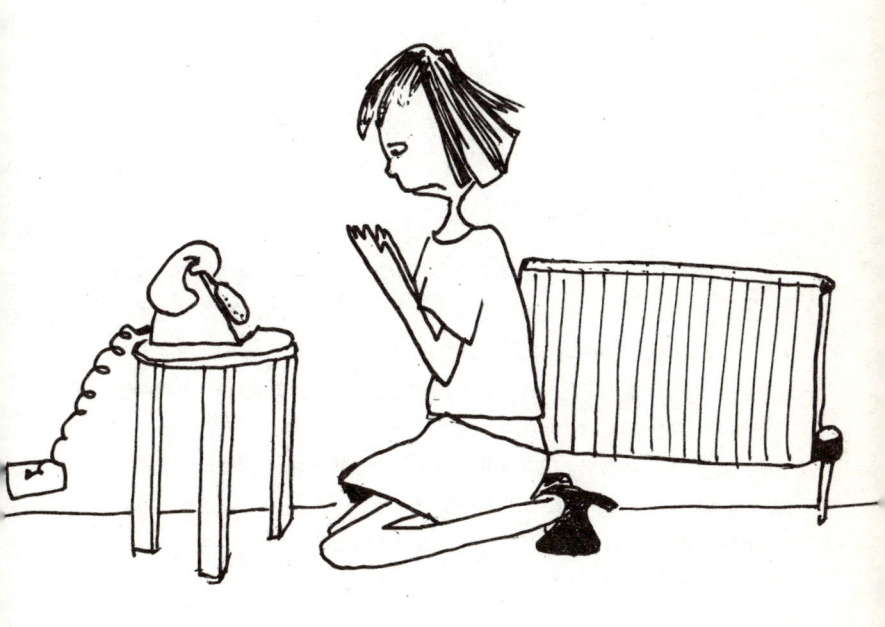

Her diary

I went to a party and met the most fantastic man tonight. He was funny, smart, and **really cute!!** His name is Jim. Isn't that the cutest name? We spent all night talking. He was interested in everything I said. Oh, and we both have the same taste in everything. *Annie Hall* is his favorite ever movie. **Just like me!** And we both really like Art Deco. And we both swim. There was just a really special connection. He took my number. I hope he calls me. I hope he calls me. **I hope he calls me!! PLEASE LET HIM CALL ME!!!!!!!!**

HIS DIARY

Went to a party. Got pretty wasted.

Her diary

Oh God, he hasn't called. It's been three days! Maybe if I hold my breath for a minute he'll call ... No, that didn't work. Asked my friend Carol and she said he'd definitely call. Maybe if I hold my breath and think of every Woody Allen movie he'll call ... No, that didn't work. Why won't he call? What's wrong with me? I really liked him. I want to be Mrs. Jim—Oh no, I don't even know his last name! **Please let him call!!** I'll do anything. I'll start doing volunteer work, I'll help people. **PLEASE!!!!!!!!!!**

HIS DIARY

I found a crumpled paper in my jacket pocket. I think it has some girl's number on it. I think I met her at that party the other night. I was so wasted.

Her diary

He called! He called! He called! He CALLED! WE'RE GOING OUT FRIDAY. HE CALLED!!!

HIS DIARY

Oh God! Called that number. She sounded insane. I think I made a date with her for Friday. Wish to God I could remember what she looked like.

Her diary

He's sooo amazing. Such a great listener. It was the best date **EVER!** He was so interested in everything I said. He was quiet but in a very cool and **VERY DEEP** way. He asked all the right questions. We kissed and it was so romantic.

HIS DIARY

Turned up to the date still hung over from the night before. She wouldn't stop talking. Couldn't get a word in. Nice tits though. Made out for a bit.

Her diary

He hasn't called! **I don't understand**—it was a perfect evening. Carol says maybe he had to go out of town. Maybe he lost my number?

HIS DIARY

Pulled an all-nighter to finish that project at work. The Boss says I did a great job.

Her diary

He still hasn't called. What's wrong with me? It's because I'm fat and hideous. No one's ever going to love me, I'm going to end up alone! Maybe he's sick? Maybe he got run over and is in a coma, and no one knows to tell me? That would be a relief. I *have* to find out!

I drove past where he lives and his lights were on, but maybe they belonged to his roommate? I'm going to go to where he works and casually bump into him, even if I have to stay there all day.

HIS DIARY

Bumped into that girl I went out with last week. We went out for a drink. She seemed kinda cute. And sexy. We had a laugh. I asked her to dinner. I'm not sure, but she seemed to like me.

Her diary

I had to pretend to be casually walking by Jim's work for five hours in the freezing rain. But I finally saw him and feigned surprise. I deserve an Oscar for Best Performance by a Stalker. I steered him toward a bar and we stayed there for hours, just talking. And the best part,

WE'RE GOING OUT AGAIN!!!!!

I *have* to get a new outfit! I saw this really great skirt; it was expensive, but now I *have* to get it. Oh, and I need new boots for it. I think I read somewhere that men like boots. And I am definitely getting my hair done. I'll have it blown super straight. I **CAN'T** wait!

HIS DIARY

Have way too much work on right now. Was going to cancel my date, but maybe it will be good to take a few hours off work. Might be fun...

Her diary

Tomorrow we will celebrate six months of being together. I'm going to cook his favorite meal. Steak with potatoes *au gratin*. And apple pie for dessert. And I've just spent a fortune on new underwear. But it is so pretty and makes my breasts look amazing. Everything is going so perfectly. I just love him so much—he's **the one**.

Mrs. Jim Brooks ... Mrs. J. Brooks ... Mr. and Mrs. J. Brooks ... Mr. and Mrs. Jim Brooks ... Jim and Susan Brooks cordially invite you to their New Year's Eve Party ... Jim and Susan Brooks invite you to their house in the Hamptons...

HIS DIARY

The scariest words a man can hear:
"Do you know what today is?"

Of course I don't know. I've just woken up and some woman starts whispering about what day it is. Luckily, I was so groggy I couldn't speak, and all I had to do was lie there and let her talk. (Which seems to happen a lot.) Apparently we've been together six months. Wow! I didn't realize it was so long. Man, she cooked a delicious dinner. And she bought some hot underwear.

Her diary

Jim woke up this morning, distracted. I couldn't get his attention. I asked him to take me to lunch, and he vaguely mentioned he had something else on. I was so worried. I had lunch with Carol. We went to that really cute place on the river. They have the most delicious salads there. I discussed Jim with her. Carol thought that maybe Jim was worried about me.

After lunch we went shopping. I bought Jim a blue sweater, which should bring out his eyes. He has such gorgeous eyes. I was late meeting him for dinner. I thought he would be mad about that, but he made no comment.

Conversation seemed so difficult, so stilted. I begged him to tell me what was wrong. What could I do to fix it? He said it had nothing to do with me. He told me not to worry.

On the way home I told him that I loved him. He simply smiled and kept driving. He didn't say "I love you, too." He just kept driving with a tight expression on his face.

When we got home I felt as if I had lost him, as if he wanted nothing to do with me anymore. He went straight to the couch and just sat there, watching TV. He seemed so distant and absent. I asked him if he wanted to talk and he just shook his head.

Finally I decided to go to bed. About ten minutes later he came to bed and to my surprise he responded to my caress and we made love, but I still felt that he was distracted and his thoughts were somewhere else.

I couldn't take it anymore, so I decided to confront him with the situation, but he had fallen asleep. I started crying and cried until I fell asleep, too.

I don't know what to do. I'm almost sure that his thoughts are with someone else. **My life is a disaster**.

HIS DIARY

My team lost the championship, but at least I got laid.

CHAPTER EIGHT

Breaking up is Hard to Do

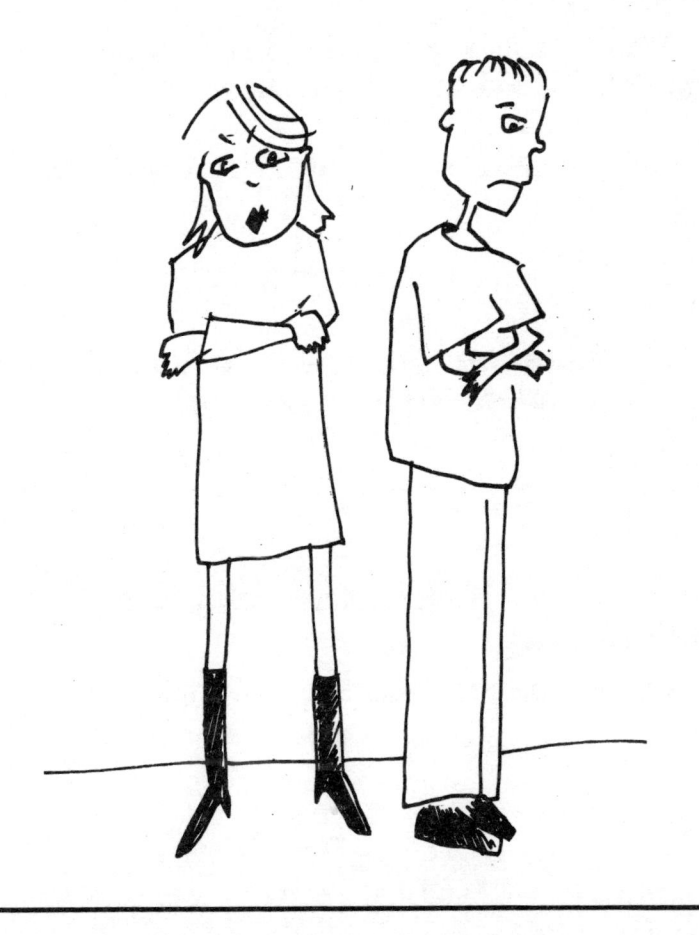

A man is sitting at home watching TV and drinking. Suddenly he hears a car screech to a halt outside and his wife rushes in, carrying a huge pile of packages and boxes.

"Pack your bags," she shouts, **"I've just won the lottery!"**

"That's unbelievable," he replies. **"Should I pack for the beach, for skiing, or what?"**

"It doesn't matter," she screams, **"just get out!"**

Question: Why is divorce so expensive?
Answer: Because it's worth it.

My husband and I divorced over **religious differences**.
He thought he was God, and I didn't.

An elderly couple decide to get a divorce. They find a lawyer and say, "We want a divorce."

The lawyer asks, "How long have you been married?"

"70 years," they proudly reply.

"70 years!" he exclaims. "And now you want to get divorced? Why on earth did you wait so long?"

The couple say, together, **"We wanted to wait until the kids were dead."**

Why do men stay in bad marriages?

Because they have no idea how to pack.

Why do women stay in bad marriages?

They have no idea how to back the car out of the garage.

Men, you know the **relationship's** over when...

She starts taping her favorites from your CD collection.

You get asked to appear on the *Jerry Springer* Show.

After six years of marriage, she says: "You didn't think we were dating exclusively, did you?"

She's started doing **volunteer work at the Fire Station**.

She sings "I Will Survive" all the time.

She's stopped wearing her ring—and started wearing her "Fuck Me I'm Single" t-shirt.

She tells you that putting all her belongings in packing crates is because it "makes the place look tidier."

When you say you want sex, **she gives you money for a prostitute**.

She's lost weight, had her hair cut, and tells you she's going on a date.

She's **shaved her head**, is wearing work boots, wants to be called Frank, and keeps taking about how much she admires Martina Navratilova and k.d. lang.

She hasn't actually come home since 1997.

Women, you know the **relationship's** over when…

He's wearing a wig and a dress, and wants to be called Sue.

You find **lipstick on his collar**—and his cock.

He's started to sleep in the spare room—of his cousin in Canada.

He tells you he's going on a long mission, deep undercover in Afghanistan—but he's a plumber.

You catch him **buying lingerie** that's far too small for you and he tells you it's so you'll have "something to aim your diet at."

He listens to Paul Simon's **"50 ways to leave your lover"**—and takes notes.

He says he loves your family … and, in particular, your sister.

He starts setting you up **on blind dates**.

He points out that the only way to recapture the excitement of the beginning of your relationship is to start a relationship with someone else.

He keeps phoning to say he'll be working late at the office, even though he works from home.

There's a **right way** and a **wrong way** to break up

For him:

Do say: It's not you, it's me.
Don't say: It's not you, it's the other woman I met.

Do say: I don't think we're physically compatible.
Don't say: Maybe if you had moved in bed once, you unresponsive bitch!

Do say: I don't think we have a future together.
Don't say: I've seen the future: your mother looks like a gargoyle—I'm scared!

Do say: We don't have any interests in common.
Don't say: You don't interest me at all.

Do say: I feel we're moving in different directions.
Don't say: I'm moving to Canada without you.

Do say: We have to talk.
Don't say: Why don't you shut up for one second so I can dump you?

Do say: I need space.
Don't say: You have half an hour to clear your crap out of my house!

Do say: It's just a trial separation.
Don't say: 'Cos otherwise I'll be on trial for your murder.

Do say: I'm not ready to make a commitment.
Don't say: I am ready to make a commitment —just not to you.

For her:

Do say: I need to concentrate on my career.
Don't say: Even my stupid dull job is more important than you.

Do say: I don't see us having a future together.
Do say: Unfortunately, I do see a future together—living in a dump with no money, loser! Get a job!

Do say: Of course there's no one else.
Don't say: Unless you count your brother, my boss, the 5th Airborne Division...

Do say: We're both looking for different things.
Don't say: I happen to be looking for someone better than you.

Do say: I feel suffocated.
Don't say: I fantasize about putting my hands around your scrawny throat and squeezing.

Do say: Let's stay friends.
Don't say: So I can torture you by describing in minute detail all the times I have sex with other men.

Do say: We're not compatible physically.
Don't say: After you, I'm definitely a lesbian for life!

Do say: There's something missing.
Don't say: A full-sized penis.

Do say: This isn't working for me.
Don't say: But my vibrator is!

Do say: This relationship isn't going anywhere.
Don't say: I'm ready to move on to the next guy who won't commit to me.

CHAPTER NINE

Growing Old Disgracefully

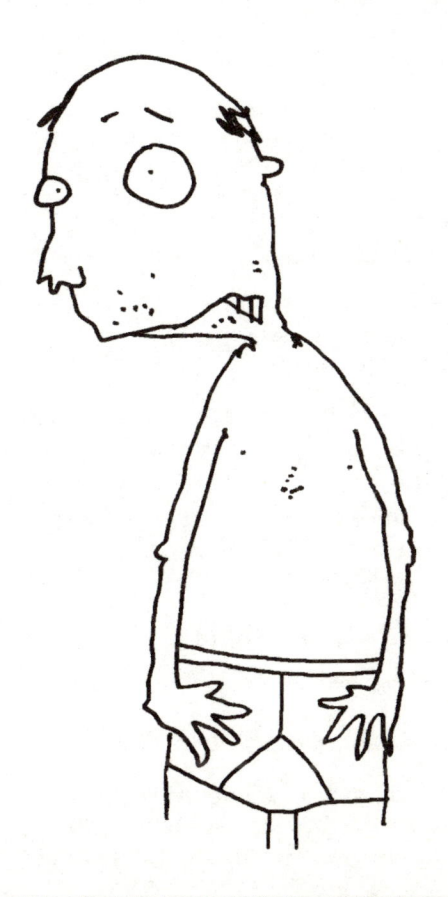

The advice column

DEAR ADVICE COLUMN,

I'VE BEEN MARRIED TO MY WIFE FOR 25 YEARS. I'M BORED AND HAVE BEEN THINKING OF ENDING THE MARRIAGE. I'M 50 AND VERY SUCCESSFUL. SHOULD I TAKE A CHANCE?

SIGNED BORED WITH MY WIFE

Dear Bored with My Wife,

Of course! You're still a relatively young man. You have time to fool around, and then you can start a whole new family with a much younger woman. We advise finding a good divorce lawyer and start hiding all your assets in offshore accounts so your wife doesn't get her greedy hands on your hard-earned wealth. Good luck with your new life!

Dear Advice Column,

My husband doesn't seem to be interested anymore. He doesn't want to sleep with me and his eyes glaze over when I talk to him. We've been married 25 years and I can't help but yearn for something more exciting. Is it too late for me?

Signed Yearning for More

Dear Yearning for More,

It's never too late. You go out there and screw the mailman, the plumber, and the video store boy. Nothing perks up a husband's interest more than having a complete slut for a wife.

A husband and wife are getting ready for bed.

The wife is standing in front of a **full-length mirror** taking a hard look at herself.

"You know sweetie," she says, "I look in the mirror and all I see is an old woman. My face is all wrinkled, my boobs are barely above my waist, and my butt is hanging out a mile. I've got huge thighs and my arms are all flabby."

She turns to her husband and says, "Tell me something **positive** to make me feel better about myself."

He thinks for a bit and then says in a soft voice, **"Well ... there's nothing wrong with your eyesight."**

How you know you're middle-aged?

For her:

1. The hair growth on your legs slows down, which gives you plenty of time to deal with your newly acquired moustache.

2. Watch those **saggy arms** when you're wearing a sleeveless shirt. If you wave goodbye to someone, you may poke your eye out.

3. When you can stand naked in front of a mirror and **you can see your bottom** without turning around.

4. When you go for a mammogram and realize that this is the only time someone will ask you to appear topless.

5. When you want to grab every firm young girl in a tube top and scream, "Listen honey, even the Roman Empire fell and those will, too!"

6. When your memory starts to go. In fact, the only thing you can retain is water.

7. Middle age means that you become more reflective ... pondering the **BIG** questions. What is life? Why am I here? What is my name again?

8. You look at your husband and think, "When did HE get old?"

For him:

1. You see a beautiful woman walking down the street and you think, mmm, she looks … **like my daughter.**

2. You pee more than you masturbate.

3. You find yourself watching **porn** and thinking: "Mmm, that bedroom is nicely furnished."

4. You have enough **pills** in your bathroom cabinet to kill every rock band in the country.

5. Your idea of a great night out is checking out your neighbor's barbecue.

6. You officially **look like an ass** in your Porsche.

7. You go to kick a football back to some kids in the park and you **need a wheelchair** for a week.

8. You look at your wife and think, "When did SHE get old?"

One morning while making breakfast, a man walked up to his wife, pinched her on the bottom, and said, **"If you got rid of this, we could get rid of your control-top pantihose."**

While she was irritated, she kept silent.

The next morning, the man woke his wife with a pinch on each of her breasts and said, **"You know, if you firmed these up, we could get rid of your bra."**

This was beyond a silent response, so she rolled over and grabbed him by the penis. With a death grip in place, she said, **"You know, if you firmed this up, we could get rid of the gardener, the postman, the poolman, and your brother!"**

A couple had been married for 40 years and also celebrated their 60th birthdays. During the celebration, **a fairy godmother** appeared and said that because they had been such a loving couple all those years, she would give them one wish each.

Being a faithful, loving spouse for all these years, naturally the wife wanted for her and her husband to have a romantic vacation together, so wished for them to travel around the world. The fairy godmother waved her hand and boom! She had the tickets in her hand.

Next, it was the husband's turn and the fairy godmother assured him he could have any wish he wanted; all he needed to do was ask for his heart's desire. He paused for a moment, then said, **"Well, honestly, I'd like to have a woman 30 years younger than me."**

The fairy godmother picked up her wand, and boom! **He was 90.**

Mrs. Ward goes to the doctor's office to collect her husband's test results.

The lab tech says to her, "I'm sorry, ma'am, but there's been a mix-up and we have a problem. When we sent the samples from your husband to the lab, the samples from another Mr. Ward were sent as well and we are now uncertain which one is your husband's. Frankly it's either **bad or terrible**."

"What do you mean?" Mrs. Ward asked.

"Well, one has tested positive for Alzheimer's and the other for AIDS. We can't tell which is your husband."

"**That's terrible!** Can we do the test over?" questioned Mrs. Ward.

"Well, it's **really expensive** and we don't like to do it more than once."

"Well, what am I supposed to do now?"

"We recommend that you drop your husband off in the middle of town. If he finds his way home, don't sleep with him!"

Jacob, aged 92, and Rebecca, aged 89, are all excited about their decision to get married. They go for a stroll to discuss the wedding and on the way they pass a drugstore. Jacob suggests they go in.

Jacob addresses the man behind the counter: "Are you the owner?"

The pharmacist answers, "Yes."

Jacob: "We're about to get married. Do you sell heart medication?"

Pharmacist: "Of course we do."

Jacob: "How about medicine for circulation?"

Pharmacist: "All kinds."

Jacob: "Medicine for rheumatism? Scoliosis?"

Pharmacist: "Definitely."

Jacob: "How about Viagra?"

Pharmacist: "Of course."

Jacob: "Medicine for memory problems, arthritis, jaundice?"

Pharmacist: "Yes, a large variety—the works."

Jacob: "What about vitamins, sleeping pills, antidotes for Parkinson's disease?"

Pharmacist: "Absolutely."

Jacob: "You sell wheelchairs and walkers?"

Pharmacist: "All speeds and sizes."

Jacob says to the pharmacist: "We'd like to use this store as our Bridal Registry."

CHAPTER ONE

And Finally ... Some Jokes to Share

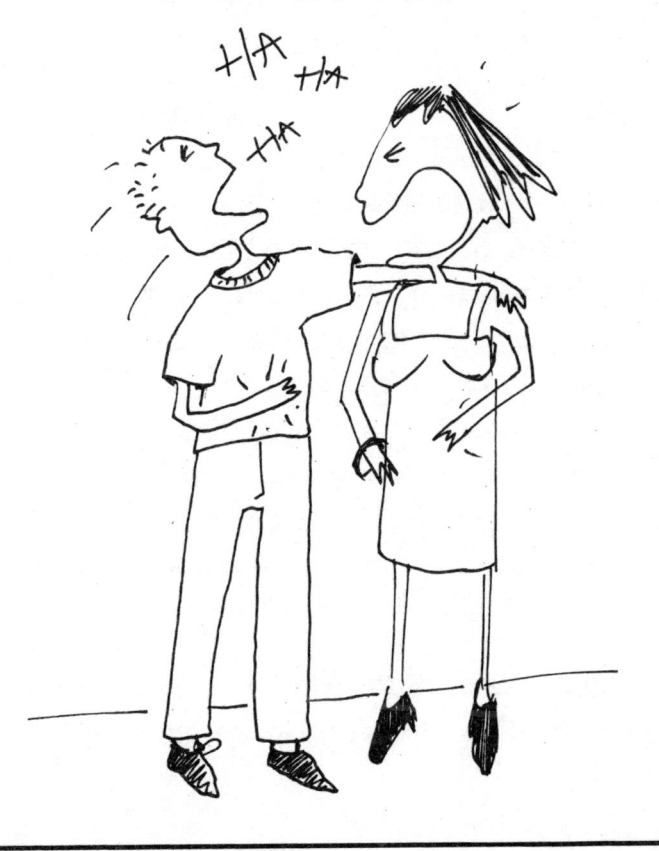

A man goes to his doctor, who tells him he has only 12 hours to live.

He goes home and tells his wife, and she holds him and comforts him, and they cry. And his wife says, **"Well, this may be your last night on Earth, but I'm going to make sure it's the best night you've ever had!"** So she puts on her sexiest clothes and cooks him his favorite meal, and they crack open a bottle of champagne, and they share a toast to the life they've had together.

Then she leads him by the hand and they make the most beautiful love they've ever had. And just as she's about to fall asleep in his arms, he says to her, **"Please, darling, just one more time. After all, this is my last night with you."** So they make love again, and again it's beautiful, and just as she's about to fall asleep in his arms, he taps her on the shoulder and says, "Once more? I love you so much and this is what I want to do most on the last night we're together." So they have sex again, and she's just about to fall asleep when he taps her on the shoulder and says, "Just once more?"

And she says, **"Sure, what do you care? You don't have to get up in the morning!"**

A man is on his deathbed and he looks up at his wife and says,

"Darling, I have to tell you something. I can't go to meet my maker with this on my conscience: I cheated on you. I cheated on you all the way through our marriage. I cheated on you with your **sister**, with your **best friend**, with **Betty** from next door, and with dozens of **other women**. All those times I was working late, or away on business trips, I wasn't: I was cheating on you!"

His wife looks placidly at him and says:

"Why do you think I poisoned your drink?"

A man was walking in the city when he was accosted by a particularly dirty and shabby-looking bum who asked him for some money for dinner. The man extracted money from his wallet and asked, "If I give you this money, will you take it and buy booze?"

"No, I stopped drinking years ago," the bum replied.

"Will you spend the money on greens fees at the golf course?"

"Are you mad? I haven't played golf in 20 years!"

The man said, "Well, I'm not going to give you money. Instead, I'm going to take you to my home for a terrific dinner cooked by my wife."

The bum was astounded. "Won't your wife be furious with you for doing that? I know I'm dirty, and probably smell pretty bad."

The man replied, **"Hey, that's ok. I just want her to see what a man looks like who's given up drink and golf."**

Tom is on his deathbed. Gathered around him are his wife and his three children. Tom looks around at his children, two of whom are cute and blond, and the eldest, Henry, who is horribly ugly and squat. Tom props himself up weakly on his pillows and says, "Kids, would you mind leaving the room for a second? I want to ask your mother something." The kids leave the room and Tom says: "Mary, please be honest with me: **am I the father of our eldest son, Henry**?"

Mary looks him in the eye and says, "Of course you are, darling. I promise you, he is absolutely yours."

Tom smiles and relaxes, lays back on his pillow and says, "Good, then I can die happy." And he dies.

Mary breathes a long sigh and says:

"Thank goodness he didn't ask about the other two..."

A man was walking across a California beach and stumbled across an old lamp. He picked it up, rubbed it, and out popped a genie.

The genie said, "OK, you released me from the lamp. You get one wish and one wish only."

The man thought about it for a while and said, "I've always wanted to go to Hawaii, but I'm afraid to fly and I get very seasick. Can you build me a bridge to Hawaii so I can drive there to visit?"

The genie laughed and replied, "That's impossible, think of the logistics of that. How would the supports ever reach the bottom of the Pacific? Think of how much concrete ... how much steel! No, think of another wish."

The man tried to think of a really good wish. Finally, he said, "I've been married and divorced four times. My wives always said that I don't care and I'm insensitive. So, I wish that I could understand women ... know how they feel inside and what they're thinking when they give me the silent treatment ... know why they're crying, know what they really want when they say 'nothing' ... know how to truly make them happy."

The genie replied, **"You want that bridge two lanes or four?"**